Just Cruising
Simple Fitness for Busy People

Sue Ward

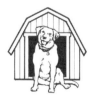

Corona House Publishing
Manhattan Beach, California

Just Cruising
Simple Fitness for Busy People

By Sue Ward

Published by:
  Corona House Publishing
  P.O. Box 398
  Manhattan Beach, CA 90267-0398
  coronahouse@earthlink.net

ISBN 0-9668104-6-5
LCCN 98-094796

Publisher's Cataloging-in-Publication
(Provided by Quality Books, Inc.)

Ward, Susan J.
     Just cruising : simple fitness for busy people /
Sue Ward. -- 1st ed.
     p. cm.
     Includes bibliographical references and index.

     1. Physical fitness. 2. Running.   I. Title.
RA781.W37 1999   613.7
                              QBI98-1693

ATTENTION FITNESS ORGANIZATIONS, PERSONAL TRAINERS AND COMMUNITY PROGRAMS:
Quantity discounts are available on bulk purchases of this book. For information, contact the publisher.

Contents

About The Author

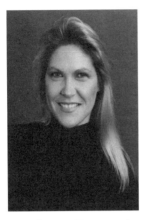

Sue Ward is the director of a large corporate fitness center in Southern California and since 1988 has worked for Health Fitness Corporation, which serves over 150 corporate clients nationwide. Sue was formerly the company's research and development coordinator and technical writer. She holds a Bachelor of Science degree in human performance and a minor in nutrition from Southern Connecticut State University. Sue has been developing fitness programs, training clients and teaching exercise classes since 1982 and holds several related certifications:

- American College of Sports Medicine
  Fitness Instructor
- American Council on Exercise
  Lifestyle & Weight Management Consultant
- American Council on Exercise
  Fitness Instructor
- Cooper Institute for Aerobics Research
  Health Promotion Director
- American Red Cross
  CPR and First Aid Instructor

Sue also serves as a member of the Program Director Committee for IDEA, the world's leading organization for health and fitness professionals. She is committed to helping people lead healthier lives through physical activity.

Acknowledgment

Many people provided valuable information and help during the development of this program and production of this book. It would be impossible to list everyone in the space provided.

First and foremost, the contributors who deserve special recognition and thanks and are among the most respected in their areas of expertise, include my editor, Paul Silva and peer reviewers, Bill Bush, Laura Liska, Brandon Flowers, Daniel Kosich, Michelle and Brian Irvine and Michelle Beale. Thank you Stacie Sakahara and Michael and Roseanne Niestemski for modeling the exercises and providing continued support and guidance.

I would also like to thank the following individuals for their contributions; Steve Reid, Ray Karimoto, Gary Horwitz, Christal Turner and my mother, Evelyn Niestemski. A very special thank you to Dan Poynter for sharing helpful information and inspiring me to complete this project and to Ken Miller, who talked me into completing my first marathon which led to the development of this program.

My clients, including my husband Donny, deserve important recognition not only for their achievements, but also for providing me with ongoing feedback which enabled me to refine the program—thank you for believing in me, the program and yourselves!

Cover by Robert Howard
Author & Chapter 6 Photos by Cheryl Ogden
Printed by Gilliland Printing

Disclaimer

This book contains the opinions and ideas of its author. It is intended to provide general information about the subject matter covered. Although the information in this book has been reviewed by sources believed to be reliable, some material may not be suited for every reader and may be affected by differences in a person's age, health, fitness level and other important factors. It is recommended you review all the available information about walking, running and general fitness and tailor the information to your individual needs.

This book is not intended to be a substitute for medical advice. Readers are strongly encouraged to consult with and receive clearance from a medical doctor before starting any fitness program or related activities. This is especially important for those who have any of the risk factors commonly associated with heart disease, which include age (over 45 years old), family history of heart disease, cigarette smoking, high blood pressure, high cholesterol, diabetes, obesity and a physically inactive lifestyle.

Every effort has been made to make this book as informative and accurate as possible; however, there may be mistakes both in typographical presentation and in content. This book should be used only as a general guide and not as the ultimate source of walking/running and fitness information. The purpose of this book is to educate and entertain. The author and Corona House Publishing shall have neither liability nor responsibility to any person or entity with respect to any loss or damage caused, or alleged to be caused, directly or indirectly by the information contained in this book.

If you do not wish to be bound by the above, you may return this book to the publisher for a full refund.

Preface

Most people believe that if you manage a fitness center, as I do, you exercise all day and are in great shape—especially if you teach a few exercise classes. The reality is that managing staff, training clients and developing programs takes up most of my time. I often find it difficult to stick to a regular workout. I consider myself moderately fit, mostly from the unstructured physical activity I get during the day.

Although I have been a fitness instructor since 1982, I have never been a runner. I only tried running a few times and always found it difficult. Once, when watching the Los Angeles Marathon on television, I was struck by two sensations: amazement, that rational people enthusiastically volunteered to run 26.2 miles, and intense curiosity about what drew the nearly 20,000 people out of bed on a Sunday morning to do it.

As a fitness professional, I realized that running is a popular fitness activity. Further, I felt I had a responsibility to my clients who asked me to provide them with running and marathon training programs. This was difficult for me since I didn't agree with the traditional, time-consuming training programs. It seemed that runners following these programs often ended up with injuries and rarely appeared to be smiling. I wanted to find a better, easier and more enjoyable way.

In 1993 I set out to develop an easy-to-follow distance running program that would be not only enjoyable, but would also focus on avoiding injuries. Being a non-runner, I was eager to develop a program for those like me who also believed this physical challenge was not possible for the "average" person.

My goal was to create a program that would help people become consistently physically active and remain motivated. Since most research cites "lack of time" as the number one reason why more people do not exercise regularly, I knew that my program also had to be realistic in terms of time commitment.

Originally, my challenge was to figure out the minimum amount of running one would have to do in order to successfully complete a marathon or half-marathon. Walking a marathon, even at a brisk 15 minute-per-mile pace could take seven or more hours and running a marathon is certainly not appealing to everyone. I searched for a more moderate and flexible approach. I searched for the compromise.

I came across some interesting training information from Jeff Galloway, a well-known Olympic runner and best-selling author, who recommends inserting walking breaks during runs—a technique he calls "Cruisin'." I respect Galloway's advice on running. He believes in smart training, proper nutrition and giving the body plenty of rest and recovery. He even recommends walking breaks for advanced runners. I went out and purchased his books on running. After using myself as a guinea pig and trying my first marathon, I decided to develop the walk/run idea into a comprehensive cruising program as a way to reach the average non-exerciser, especially those who *think* they can't run.

What I learned from developing this program was that cruising can make physical activity goals achievable. Whether you want to get fit, try a short fun run or complete a marathon, you don't have to be young or in great shape. I have trained a variety of clients. So far, all have been successful achieving their goals. Most were non-runners or people who might occasionally jog a couple of miles. Some of my clients had minor physical limitations such as knee or back problems, while others were overweight or physically inactive. The one thing all my clients had in common was the willingness to try and desire to persevere.

You'll meet many of my clients as you read this book. I wanted to share their experiences, as they are inspiring stories of success. Perhaps by hearing about where others started and what their struggles were, you too will become inspired and realize that you can do it—if you cruise it.

1
What is Cruising?
Defining the Experience

cruise /kru:z/ -v. 2b. to move
or proceed, speedily, smoothly
or effortlessly

Merriam Webster's
Collegiate Dictionary
Tenth Edition

Joyce swore she was unable to run. It was hard enough for her to start walking regularly. At 48, she was trying to lose some weight. I sensed her determination when she enrolled, for the second time, in my weight management course at the corporate fitness center where I serve as director. One day while teaching a session about exercise, I told the class I could train any "non-runner" for a half-marathon. Joyce's curiosity was piqued as she wondered if someone her age, who is overweight and lacking the time to exercise, could complete such a physical challenge.

She looked at me with a mix of disbelief and curiosity. "Do you really think I could do... how many miles is that, thirteen?" she said and then asked for a copy of my training program. "I just want to look at it," she said.

Four months later, Joyce came into the fitness center and asked for the San Diego Half-Marathon race application. Knowing that she was now walking regularly, I handed her the application and said, "I'm so glad you decided to try this. There are plenty of people who walk the whole half-marathon." She had a gleam in her eye as she told me she had been secretly following my program. "I won't be walking the whole thing. I'm up to about ten minutes of running," she said proudly.

One week later, as Joyce crossed the finish line of her first half-marathon, she experienced a tremendous sense of achievement. As a finisher's medal was placed around her neck, she looked at her family, caught her breath, wiped a tear and said, "I have not felt this great in years."

When the Tortoise Meets the Hare

Among people who exercise, there are walkers and there are runners. Walking is often viewed as an easy workout for those who are out of shape—a good place to start. It is a simple, natural activity that just about anybody can do. There is no question that walking is a great exercise; however, many who promote it tend to steer people away from running.

Running is often perceived as a strenuous activity that is hard on the body. It is a form of exercise that stirs up images of lean forms with serious faces running all over town, sometimes battling injuries. Some feel that to be considered a "real" runner, one must achieve a certain pace or complete long distances without walking. Therefore, it is common for most non-exercisers to reject the idea of running before ever giving it a try. Walking and running are generally considered separate activities for two different groups of people, who would rarely be seen exercising together. Walkers and runners seem to be worlds apart.

Now imagine these two worlds merging. A new mode of exercise is born—walk-running or "cruising." Although many fitness experts recommend cruising, especially when beginning a running program, it is rare that the combination of these two activities is the focus of attention. Cruising brings the worlds of walking and running together and can make a workout personal, fun and comfortable for your body. Think of it as a healthy compromise.

Cruising provides you with a simple, time-efficient way to be physically active, whether you are exercising for fitness or training for a marathon. With cruising, you are in control. You can choose to do mostly walking and a little running, an equal combination of the two or you can follow an easy progression that can transform the average, busy non-exerciser into a recreational runner.

Cruising is Easy

If you go outside and walk to the corner, jog across the street, then walk to the next corner, you are cruising. It's that easy. When you start the Base Training Program presented in this book, you begin with walking and gradually insert a few minutes of slow, easy running. You alternate intervals of walking and running until you complete a certain distance. The program instructs you to begin slowly and helps you to progress gradually until you establish your own "cruising plan," that is, the minutes in each run and walk interval. At the end of the Base Training Program, you may discover that you enjoy a certain cruise plan, find it possible to progress to three miles of running without any walking, or your workout may end up being mostly walking. The key to successful cruising is finding out what works best for you and what is comfortable for your body. It is also important to understand that since all bodies are different, not everyone will progress at the same rate.

Cruising Benefits

There are many health benefits of regular exercise. In nearly every fitness book or article, there are reminders about how exercise can help you lose and keep off excess body fat, lower blood pressure and cholesterol, improve circulation, sleep more soundly, boost self-esteem, elevate mood, tone muscles, increase energy and strengthen the body's immune system. The list goes on and on. Since cruising promotes regular, moderate exercise, you can expect to achieve many of these health benefits.

Cruising also offers some unique benefits:

- It is easier on your body than running which may reduce your risk of injury and allow you to go farther without becoming excessively tired

- It allows plenty of time for your joints (hips, knees, ankles) to get used to some running which may help make them stronger and well-prepared for training outdoors

- It burns more calories than walking

- You can get a good workout in a short time

- It makes learning to run seem effortless

- It can be done anywhere (even on vacation)

- It puts you in control of each workout

What Makes Cruising Different?

It requires a minimal time commitment. Lack of time is one of the main reasons why more people do not exercise regularly. Busy work schedules and family obligations prevent many from fitting exercise into their day. The Base Training program requires between 15 and 30 minutes, three days a week. For most people, this usually means two days during the week and one day on the weekend. Even if your goal is a marathon, the only additional time required for training occurs on the weekend. This is realistic for most people and is what makes cruising attractive.

It is simple, but effective. There are numerous books telling us to simplify our lives, yet many experts often make health and fitness too complex. You do not need any experience with exercise to make this program work for you. The guidelines are easy to follow and designed to keep you motivated. Even the strength and stretching programs are so simple, you may question their effectiveness; however, once you experience the amazing results, you'll be a believer in simplicity.

It is easy on the body. The slow, gradual progression and recommendations for establishing your run/walk intervals allow your body plenty of time to adapt to cruising, even if you *think* you can't run. A few minutes of slow, easy running is achievable for almost anybody, depending on your level of motivation. As you progress through the program, fitness will follow as your heart, lungs, muscles, bones and joints become stronger. You will find your own personal level of comfort with the exercise; one that won't leave you breathless.

It is designed to be enjoyable. Fun is often missing from exercise programs. If you can make exercise fun, you will be more likely to make it a permanent part of your lifestyle. The word "cruising" even sounds a bit more relaxed and enjoyable than words like "running," "walking," or "run/walk." There are a few reasons why cruising can be more fun:

- It encourages exercising outdoors
- It encourages exercising with a partner or a small group of friends
- The program is flexible

For anyone who likes being outdoors, cruising in a place where the surroundings are pleasant may be more enjoyable than working out on a treadmill in a crowded gym or at home where there can be many distractions.

Walking and running outdoors is natural to your body, unlike exercising on a treadmill which usually takes some getting used to. Also, an outdoor workout may be a better choice if you want to relieve stress. Imagine cruising along a beach at sunset, or in a beautifully landscaped park, or in your favorite neighborhood. The more you enjoy your surroundings, the more you will enjoy cruising.

Finding a workout partner or a small group of friends can also help make your workout more enjoyable and keep you motivated. Many people find that having to meet someone at a certain time strengthens their commitment to the workout. It can be fun to catch up with friends on the latest gossip, work out problems or talk about movies. It's the perfect program for married couples since it can be an opportunity to spend some quality time together. But if you are one who prefers to exercise alone, cruising can also offer a chance at solitude; time to think, relieve stress, appreciate nature and come up with new ideas to help you deal with life's challenges.

The cruising program is flexible and can be done anywhere. You may choose to take the kids along on their bikes or roller-skates. Push small children in a special stroller made for running. Take the dog along and you'll also make his day. No matter where you are, you can cruise. If you feel like running more on a particular day, you'll be able to do so. If you feel like walking, you'll be trained for that too. If you like to hike, you can do some easy running during level parts of the trail. With cruising, it is your choice, according to how you feel. You could be a walker one day and a runner the next. When you're cruising you can simply kick back, go at your own pace and enjoy.

It increases self-confidence. Since many people perceive running as a strenuous exercise, they think only young, lean, athletic types can and should run. This is simply not true. Even if you are older, overweight and have never exercised regularly, you will be able to do some slow, easy running. The key is finding the amount that you feel is comfortable.

The single most important thing you will learn after completing one or all of the cruising programs in this book is that you can do just about anything in life you choose, if you go about it one step at a time, stay committed and believe in yourself. Imagine how confident you might feel if you completed a half-marathon (that's 13.1 miles!). Cruising makes a goal like this achievable. In fact, in most large marathons, it is the *ordinary* people (or extraordinary, when it comes to commitment), not the elite runners, who make up the highest percentage of participants.

Confidence also comes from being able to stick to an exercise program. Because the cruising programs in this book are simple, require a minimal time commitment and can be done anywhere, you will find it easier to keep up with the workouts. If you consider yourself a non-runner and try the Base Training program, you will feel more confident with each workout, which helps to keep you motivated.

Cruising is Natural

I can't even say the word. I have to spell it. Whenever I ask my dog Harper if he wants to go for a w-a-l-k, he responds with an enthusiastic "woof" and sometimes a spin. He can barely keep still. Just the thought of going outdoors is exciting. So I grab the leash and we head for the park.

Harper is well-trained, so once we get there, I let him off the leash. He starts out running in any direction, enjoying the open space and fresh air. You can see how hard he's smiling (yes, dogs do smile). He slows down, walks a bit, observes his surroundings, sniffs the fresh the air and then he's off running again. He always enjoys himself so much, especially when other dogs are around. Harper, like most dogs, will rarely reject the opportunity for some outdoor physical activity.

How do you think Harper would do on a treadmill? Or a stair climbing machine? I don't think he'd be smiling quite as much. If I said to him, "Harper, would you like to workout on the treadmill?" he probably wouldn't budge. In fact, I think he'd find it quite boring and unnatural. It may sound a bit silly, but observing dogs can teach us some important things about physical activity:

- You don't mind it when it is fun

- It's usually more fun outdoors

- It's more comfortable to go at your own pace than it is someone else's (this is why Harper prefers being off the leash)

- It's easier and more enjoyable when you are with others

When given the chance, dogs naturally know how to get and stay fit. They are born cruisers.

Cruising is natural. After all, the human body was designed for forward movement. Cruising is a form of exercise that won't leave you breathless. You set the pace, naturally. From non-exercisers, to walkers, to runners who want to "get back into" their routine, cruising offers something for everyone.

How to Use This Book

This book offers three cruising programs:
    1. Base Training (6 weeks)

2. Half-Marathon (12 weeks)
3. Marathon (24 weeks)

The programs are designed to be completed in order; however, after the Base Training Program, you may decide that is enough for you. Many of my clients continue to cruise three miles, three times a week, which is realistic and time-efficient. Others gradually build their mileage by adding a half or full mile on the weekend until they reach six miles. Then they are ready to enter a 10K (a 6.2 race or fun run).

If you are pleased with your activity and fitness levels achieved through the Base Training Program, skip to the chapters on strength training and stretching to learn safe and effective exercises you can do at home. Chapter 6, "Getting Strong," shows you how to create your own muscle-conditioning workout and explains how to change it regularly. And be sure to remember to stretch, as shown in Chapter 7. A stronger and more flexible body makes cruising even easier.

Many of my clients have found the Base Training program so easy, they were inspired to try the half-marathon or marathon training programs. Chapters 4, and 5 describe each of these programs in detail and show how easy it can be for anyone to achieve these goals.

If you want to learn the basics of good nutrition or weight loss, Chapter 8 presents a simple way to improve your eating habits and lose weight (if necessary) during the program. You will learn a sensible, week-by-week approach to healthy eating, helpful tips for weight loss and what to eat before, during and after your workouts.

Chapter 9, "Cruising Q & A," should answer most other questions you have about the program. Each time I trained a new group of cruisers, I kept track of the most commonly asked questions. This chapter provides the answers.

Cruising Can Change Your Life

You've met Joyce. At 48, she cruised her first half-marathon. A year later, she did it again with her daughter Jamie who was inspired by her mother's achievement. It was Jamie's first half-marathon.

After three half-marathons, Joyce took the next step and set a new goal: cruising the Los Angeles Marathon as a way to celebrate her 50th birthday. Jamie wanted in on the challenge. So they continued training for their first marathon.

On the morning of the 1998 Los Angeles Marathon, we assembled at the Start line. Joyce's face was glowing with excitement. Here she was, standing in the middle of about 20,000 runners. She never imagined herself in this scene before. It was a perfect day, in spite of all the bad weather Southern California was experiencing that year. The gun went off and we started on our journey through Los Angeles.

Joyce's first surprise (organized by Jamie who was a few minutes ahead of us) came at mile three where she saw a crowd in blue T-shirts cheering her on. About 20 of her family members and friends proudly wore the T-shirts that read "Go Joyce!" on the front and "50 Years and 26.2 miles later..." on the back. She beamed with pride as we ran by.

We spotted Joyce's cheering team again at mile 13 and at mile 20, loudly making their presence known to those passing by. Each time we came upon her "birthday partiers," as we began to call them, they would drive to the next planned cheering spot, staying one step ahead of us. Several times, I heard runners say, "Who is Joyce?" The support for Joyce by her family and friends was tremendous. It helped propel her to the marathon finish line.

Later that evening, I was invited to Joyce's post-race, 50th birthday party. The cake, the napkins, the poster, everything read:

"50 years and 26.2 miles later ..."

Jamie had planned a great party for her mother, nearly forgetting that she too had run her first marathon that day. Joyce stood before her family and friends thanking everyone for the support. "My cousin jumped out of a plane on her 50th birthday and since I've always been somewhat competitive with her — I just had to do this," she said. Jamie presented Joyce with the family gift. "This is not just a victory celebration, it's my mom's special birthday. We are so proud of you, not just as a marathoner, but as a mother." Jamie then placed a solid gold Los Angeles Marathon medal around her mom's neck. The inscription on the back read:

"Living an ordinary life, in an extraordinary way"

I too was proud of Joyce. Some people become depressed as birthdays approach, others choose to celebrate life! You could say cruising changed Joyce's life. It could change yours too. Anything is possible!

2
Cruising Essentials
What You Need Before You Start

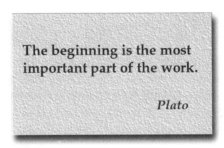

> The beginning is the most important part of the work.
>
> *Plato*

To get the most out of this program, it is important to be prepared. Follow the simple steps described in this chapter; they hold the key to your success.

Health Screening

Consult your primary care physician before beginning this exercise program, especially if you have health issues such as smoking, high blood pressure, high cholesterol, diabetes, obesity, family history of heart disease or a physically inactive lifestyle. If you take medications, ask your doctor how they might affect your workout. Share the cruising program and its philosophy with your doctor, who will be pleased you have decided to take a positive step toward better health.

Set a Goal

Goals provide focus and help you to evaluate your progress. They keep your challenge clear and provide ongoing motivation. Think about what you want to get out of the program and write it down. This is your goal. Use the tips below to help refine and clarify your goal.

Be Specific Set goals that are specific and measurable. Instead of setting a goal to "get in better shape by trying the cruising program," set a more specific goal such as to cruise three days a week for three weeks and improve your one-mile time by 30 seconds. To measure this goal, you can time yourself during the first workout and again after the ninth workout to see how you have improved your time.

Be Realistic Set goals that are realistic, but challenging. If you have never stuck to an exercise program, do not set a goal to cruise three days a week, do strength training three days a week and improve your eating habits. A more realistic goal would be to cruise three days a week for the first three weeks. Then, after you achieve that goal, set a new goal and gradually incorporate other aspects of the program.

Time It If you start by setting short-term goals, such as the examples above, you will be more likely to stay motivated. Shorter or longer time periods may be applied. If you have long-term goals in mind, great. Remember they are achieved by taking small steps.

This book presents three goal-oriented cruising programs: Base Training, Half-Marathon and Marathon Training. Each is described in subsequent chapters. It is not overly-ambitious to want to eventually try a marathon. That might be your long-term goal; however, start with the Base Training Program. It is intended for those who are not physically active and those who think they can't run. After completion of the 6-week program, you will be cruising three times a week for three miles during each workout. At that point, evaluate the program. If you like cruising, keep going. Try adding one mile to your weekend cruise for the next three weeks or try the Half-Marathon program next. You'll be amazed at how easy it is to achieve your goals when you take small steps.

Set Your Schedule

Make a commitment to cruise three days a week. Pick the days and times that work best with your current lifestyle. Any days you choose are fine, just be sure to leave at least one day of rest between workouts. To be successful, you must commit to your schedule. You can be flexible, but it is important to complete the workouts.

Do not cruise more than three days a week. If you want to do more activity on your "off" days, choose other low impact activities such as walking, biking, roller-skating, swimming or exercise classes. Whatever activities you select, be sure they are ones you enjoy.

Find the Perfect Location

Training outdoors will give you the best results, especially if it is your goal to cruise a road race. Look for a relatively flat walking path along a beach, lake front or in a park. Training on concrete is acceptable, as long as the surface is level. Cruising on city streets is not recommended since cars, noise and pollution are unpleasant, especially if one of your goals is to decrease stress.

When selecting a training location, try to find a place where you can cruise a total of three miles. It is also helpful to know where each mile mark is so you can see your improvements as you progress through the program. Many of my clients have used a bicycle with an odometer to measure the distances where they train. If you don't know the distances where you are training, you can follow the same cruising programs based on time (see Appendix).

You may train indoors on a treadmill, if it works best with your lifestyle and climate. Treadmill cruising works well for those who simply want to get and stay fit. But if your goal includes cruising a road race, it is important to complete at least one workout per week outdoors since the training is more specific to your goal. Outdoor cruises, which are all human-powered, are not only more challenging, they help to establish your cruising pace.

Invest in a Pair of Running Shoes

Even if your cruising workout consists mostly of walking, buy a good pair of running shoes. This way, if you decide to do more running, you will be prepared. Choose a shoe that is comfortable and fits properly. Some experts recommend buying the shoes a half or full size larger than your normal shoe size, especially if you are training long distances. This is because your feet can swell during training and cause discomfort or injury. Other experts say to ensure a proper fit, there should be a thumbnail's width between the tips of your shoe and your big toe. Either way, it is important the shoes fit.

For help with shoe selection, go to a reputable, "runner's" store and seek the help of an experienced salesperson (preferably a runner). Tell the salesperson your goal and training plan. If you have a history of hip, knee or ankle injuries, your shoe could be the key to injury prevention. Sometimes, you have to try different brands before you find the one that is right for your foot. One good way to select a comfortable running shoe is to get about 10 pairs of running shoes, then put different models on each foot. Keep the more comfortable shoe on. Put the next shoe on. You can end up with a good shoe by using a simple process of elimination. Keep track of the miles you put on your running shoes; most should give you 500 to 600 miles before the cushioning wears down.

Shoe Tip

For help with selecting a running shoe, call the American Running and Fitness Association (ARFA) at 800-776-ARFA or visit their web site at **www.arfa.org** and ask them to mail you a copy of *Beat the Choosing Your Running Shoes Blues*. This brochure offers tips for choosing a shoe that is right for you. For $10, you can fill out a questionnaire, take a few simple foot tests and mail your form back to ARFA to be entered into their running shoe database. After you send back the form you will receive a printout of running shoes that match your needs. This service is free to members of ARFA or members of the American Medical Athletic Association. This service may be a good starting point, after which you can rely on experience.

While you are at the store, buy a few pairs of running socks. They do make a difference. Look for a sock that has extra cushioning in the ball of the foot, toes and heel area. Choose a brand that is made of a fabric that keeps moisture away from the skin. As with your shoes, be sure the socks fit and always try on running shoes with your running socks.

Select Comfortable Clothing

Just about anything comfortable will do if you are cruising for short periods of time. I sometimes wear jeans and a T-shirt when I go for a quick cruise with my dog. For regular workouts, standard exercise clothing is best. Supportive running tights or bike shorts with a T-shirt is my favorite outfit since it is light and comfortable. On cool days, wear a sweatshirt over your T-shirt. On hot days, a tank top will keep you cool. If you are considering a half or full marathon, your clothing choices become more important (see Chapter 4).

Log Your Workouts

Since cruising involves running and walking intervals, you will need a watch with a stopwatch feature or a digital watch to time the intervals. Many runner's watches have interval timers, so you can preset your cruising plan while also monitoring your total time.

Tracking your cruising workouts is a great way to stay motivated. This book provides training schedules on which you can record your cruising time and mileage. Some people prefer noting workouts on a wall calendar. Others like to write in a journal or daily planner. Be sure to make notations about the weather, what you ate, etc.. Your tracking log is the way you will see improvements and learn what works and what doesn't work for you.

Brett, one of my clients, entered his workouts into a spreadsheet in the computer. Each time we went out for a cruise, he noted the mileage, time and weather. After finishing his first marathon, he gave me the log and summed up all the miles we ran since starting the program. It was amazing to see those totals!

Find a Workout Partner

When I first developed the cruising programs, I did all of my training alone. That was not easy, but I had some pleasant surroundings and enjoyed experiencing some solitude. I cruised along the beach in Southern California, listening to the waves crash, breathing the fresh sea air and often watching beautiful sunsets. Now I have several workout partners who keep me motivated. I cruise sometimes with my husband, a former non-exerciser. I trained him for his first marathon and crossing the finish line together was a magical moment. Each year I train a small group of new exercisers and make plans to meet them every Saturday morning. I also cruise with my dog, who can never talk me out of it. Finding a work-out partner can make the difference between sticking to a program and giving up.

Nutrition

Be sure your body is well-nourished at all times. This means eating a balanced diet which should include whole grains, fruits and vegetables as the foundation. As you will learn later in Chapter 8, "Nutrition and Weight Loss," making small and gradual changes in your eating habits is the best way to improve nutrition and lose weight (if necessary). Dieting will only make you feel weak and deprived and is *not* part of the cruising program. If you are eager to improve your eating habits, set some short-term goals. Here are a few examples:

- Avoid snacks after dinner three days a week

- Make two meals a week consist of nothing but fruits and vegetables

- Switch from soda (diet or regular) to natural juice beverages or water

- Reduce portions at one meal every day

- Switch from white breads to 100% whole grain breads

Keep in mind, regular exercise does not correct poor eating habits.

Follow The Cruising Guidelines

Always follow the six cruising guidelines to help make sure your workout is safe and effective. You will be reminded of these guidelines again as you read through each of the three cruising programs. Memorize them and during your workouts ask yourself if you are following the guidelines, especially if you experience any difficulty with the program.

1. Commit to three days a week; no more, no less.

Cruising more than three days a week may increase you chance of injury and decrease your level of commitment. Remember, the goal here is a time-efficient exercise program that will fit into your busy lifestyle. If you cruise less than three days a week, you may successfully achieve your goals, but it will take longer. Three out of seven days is realistic, moderate and works.

2. Always warm up and cool down.

The best warm-up and cool-down for any activity is to do that activity, but at a low intensity. Begin each cruise with three to five minutes of walking. Start slowly and work up to a brisk walking pace or a light jog. If your body feels tight, stretch briefly, but only after the three to five-minute warm-up. Muscles and joints that are warm are better-prepared for exercise and less likely to become injured.

To cool down, end every cruise by walking for 5-10 minutes. Longer cruises require a longer cool-down; at least 15-20 minutes. Start your cool-down by walking briskly and progress to a slower pace. Conclude your cool-down session with 10-15 minutes of stretching, especially if you want to maintain or improve your flexibility (see Chapter 7).

3. Use good form.

Good running and walking form can make your workout easier. Always maintain an upright posture. Keep your shoulders and arms relaxed and close to your body. When running, keep your feet close to the ground and "run quietly." I usually tell my clients, "if you can hear your feet landing, you are running too hard." Run and walk heel-to-toe and breathe deeply. If your breathing becomes too difficult, check to be sure your chest is forward and posture tall. If all this is too much to think about, concentrate on one tip at a time and when in doubt, do what feels most comfortable and natural to you.

4. Take water breaks.

Proper water intake is important. If water is not available where you are cruising, then carry a water bottle that fits easily into the palm of your hand. This way you can take frequent sips which may help the water to be better absorbed by your body and may also be more comfortable for your stomach. Be sure to drink water before, during and after your workout. On hot days or during long cruises, you must increase your water breaks. (See Chapter 8 for specific guidelines about fluid intake.)

5. Be flexible.

Lack of sleep, inadequate nutrition or fluid intake, illness, climate or environment can affect your workout. It is a fact of exercise that some days will be harder than others. Recognize when you are having a hard day and ease up by including longer walking intervals or by shortening your workout for that day. On days when you are feeling strong, you may want to try longer running intervals or a faster pace. Remember, cruising workouts are flexible.

6. Keep a positive attitude.

Nothing is more powerful than believing you can achieve your goals. Be proud of your accomplishments after every workout. You are taking steps to improve your health and well-being. Tell yourself how amazing you are! This is especially important on those days when the workout feels tough. If you have a cruising partner or group, avoid complaining about personal problems unless it helps you relieve stress and come up with solutions. Talk about the happiest moments in your life, great movies or funny stories. Keep focused on your short-term goal. You are strong. You can do it!

Now You Are Ready To Cruise

You are on your way. All you have left to do is pick a starting day and mark it on your calendar. In a few weeks you will be telling others about your accomplishments. Be prepared to impress your friends and family and inspire others. Enjoy the cruise!

3
Building a Base
Cruising For Fun, Fitness or Your First Short Race

> Generally speaking, all parts of the body which
> have a function, if used in moderation and
> exercised in labors to which each is accustomed,
> becomes thereby healthy and well-developed,
> and age slowly; but if unused and left to idle,
> they become liable to disease, defective in growth,
> and age quickly.
>
> *Hippocrates*

Norma ran sporadically, but quickly became worn out and discouraged after only a few minutes into each workout. After hearing about the cruising program from a coworker, she decided to give it a try. I suggested the Base Training Program, but since she was unable to maintain proper running form, I was not sure if she would be successful. She ran with her hips turned out, landing on her toes, with her feet pointing outward. I was concerned that this might increase her chances of injury, so I worked with her and tried to correct her form. The attempt was unsuccessful.

For 40 years, Norma has walked with her hips turned out. So I decided to stop trying to correct that which was comfortable and completely natural to her and proceeded to guide her through the Base Training Program. Not only did she complete the six-week program, but she gained the confidence to train for and finish her first half-marathon six months later. She credits her injury-free accomplishment to the slow, gradual progression recommended in the Base Training Program.

Start Out Right

The Base Training Program is a six-week introduction to cruising. It is designed to:

- Provide a simple, moderate, time-efficient exercise program that will improve your level of physical conditioning

- Help your body slowly adapt to a combination of running and walking

- Help you identify a run/walk combination that you find comfortable and enjoyable

- Offer an injury-free way to start a running program

- Increase your self-confidence

The Base Training Program uses easy run/walk combinations to guide you through a gradual progression in time and distance. You begin by alternating two minutes of running and three minutes of walking until you reach a total distance of one mile. For most people, this first workout takes between 12 and 16 minutes, which is a realistic and moderate starting point. You repeat this workout three times before increasing distance or running minutes. By week six, you will have identified a run/walk combination that works best for you or, if you follow the program precisely, it is likely you will be able to run three miles (without any walking), three times a week.

What is a "Cruise Plan?"

A "cruise plan" is a term I use to identify a run/walk combination. For example, a 2:3 cruise plan means you alternate two minutes of running and three minutes of walking until you reach your distance goal. As you progress through the Base Training Program, you will notice the cruise plan changing to reflect a gradual increase in the length of the run intervals. The distance also increases by a half-mile each week. In the last two weeks of the program, the walk interval decreases from three to two minutes. If your goal is to be able to run three miles without walking, try it at the end of the sixth week. Chances are you will be able to do it!

The Base Training Program

	Day One *run:walk* *(minutes)*	Day Two *run:walk* *(minutes)*	Weekend *run:walk* *(minutes)*
Week 1 *1 mile*	2:3	2:3	2:3
Week 2 *1.5 miles*	3:3	4:3	5:3
Week 3 *2 miles*	6:3	7:3	8:3
Week 4 *2.5 miles*	10:3	12:3	14:3
Week 5 *3 miles*	15:2	15:2	15:2
Week 6 *3 miles*	20:2	25:2	Try to run 3 miles without walking!

Column one shows the distance goal for each week of the program. The remaining columns show the cruise plan for each workout. The program may feel easy at first for some people and difficult for others. Remember, everyone is different and how you progress may be affected by several contributing factors:

- current level of activity
- body type and weight (heavier bodies adapt more slowly)
- level of motivation
- history of injury

Keep in mind, the heart and lungs adapt more quickly to exercise than the muscles, bones and joints. So, even if you find the program easy at times, stay with the slow and gradual progression; it is the key to cruising and injury prevention. It also helps prevent you from becoming breathless during your workouts which makes cruising more enjoyable.

How to Modify the Program

If it's too hard...

Little aches and pains are normal as your body adapts to the exercise, but if you find the program too difficult, go back to the previous cruise plan and repeat it for at least three workouts. After three workouts, you should be ready to move on; however, if you feel you have reached your limit in terms of running minutes, then simply stay with that cruise plan and follow the program to your distance goal. This is how to identify your personal cruise plan.

James, a busy 52 year-old executive who never tried running, had some trouble working through the Base Training Program. At six feet, four inches tall, 255 pounds, and with a history of knee and back injuries, he realized the progression was too hard on his body. Once he reached a 7:3 cruise plan, he felt he had reached his limit in running minutes. He continued to progress in distance and experimented with shorter walking intervals. For fitness, James now cruises three miles, three times a week and settled on a 7:1 cruise plan. Be sure to modify the program to fit your needs and level of comfort.

If it's too easy... If you are already exercising regularly and have some experience with running, you may not need to start with the Base Training Program. Where you start depends on your fitness level, ability to run, history of injury, body weight and current exercise schedule. Most people who have some experience with running can start at Week 3, but keep in mind that starting off easier gives your body more time to adapt which may be a better way to prevent injuries down the road.

Record Your Cruise

After each workout, make some notes about the cruise and how you felt. Evaluate your breathing, the way your muscles and joints felt, how your feet felt, your level of enjoyment and your sense of accomplishment. When you look back at your notes after six weeks, you'll be surprised to learn what started out as somewhat challenging is now quite easy.

Record the total amount of time it takes to complete the distance goal, not including your warm-up and cool-down. This will help you identify your per mile pace and help show your improvements. To find your per mile pace, divide the total time by the distance.

EXAMPLE: Let's say you are in Week 3 and using a 6:3 cruise plan. It took you 25 minutes and 30 seconds to complete a distance of 2 miles.

25.5 (twenty-five and a half minutes) / 2 (miles)
= 13.25 (thirteen and a quarter minutes)
or 13 minutes and 15 seconds per mile

Write your per-mile pace on your chart as **13:15**.

Remember the Cruising Essentials and Guidelines

Michelle, a busy housewife who rarely exercised, initially had some trouble following the program and was about to give up after only a few weeks. Others in her cruising group seemed to move effortlessly through the workouts to each new level. After missing a few workouts, she became discouraged, which affected her overall attitude. When Michelle went back and reviewed the cruising guidelines, she realized she was not following four of the six guidelines. Accepting the fact that it may take her longer than six weeks because she was missing workouts, not drinking enough water and had not exercised in many years, she was able to make some changes and continue at her own pace.

If you finish a workout and feel discouraged, ask yourself if you are missing any of the cruising essentials and if you are following the guidelines (see Chapter 2).

Cruising Guidelines

1. **Cruise three days a week; no more, no less.**

2. **Always warm up and cool down.**

3. **Use good form.**

4. **Take water breaks.**

5. **Be flexible.**

6. **Keep a positive attitude.**

Keep Cruising!

Once you have completed the Base Training Program and have experienced cruising, you have several options for continuing with a time-efficient, moderate exercise program:

- Stay with your goal of cruising three times a week for fun or fitness.

- To stay motivated and to celebrate your accomplishment, walk, run or cruise a 5K road race (3.1 miles).

- Be a walker or runner during the week and a cruiser on the weekends.

- Add some quick and easy strength training exercises (see Chapter 6).

- Try cruising during a hike; running on level ground and walking up the hills.

- Take the family or the dog out for regular short cruises.

- Continue training and set a new goal; a 10K road race (6.2 miles) or proceed to the Half-Marathon Cruising Program (you can do it; cruising makes it possible).

How to Train For a 10K

If you completed the Base Training Program, you can be ready for a 10K in 3-6 weeks. Simply add a half or full mile to your weekend cruise every week until you reach six miles. Keep your weekday workouts to three miles. Use this same general rule when training for any race up to 10 miles.

Remember, with cruising you can be a walker or a runner. Your body will be trained for each or a combination of these activities. You have a choice with each workout.

Resource Recommendations

Keep yourself motivated by learning more about your exercise options. There are a variety of resources that present different ways of fitting fitness into a busy life and expand on the information presented in this chapter.

The Complete Idiot's Guide to Jogging and Running by Bill Rodgers with Scott Douglas—Alpha Books, New York, NY

> **Comments:** I love this book! It's fun to read and geared toward the novice. It is a complete reference to running, explained in the easiest terms. There are so many fun facts in this book, you'll never get tired of reading.

Galloway's Book on Running by Jeff Galloway
Shelter Publications, Inc., Bolinas, CA

> **Comments:** This is an excellent running reference. In it you can learn how to take your training to the next level by following the advice of former Olympian Jeff Galloway. He was among the first to promote cruising!

Fitness For Dummies™ by Suzanne Schlosberg and Liz Neporent—IDG Books Worldwide, Inc., Foster City, CA

> **Comments:** This is an excellent reference book, which covers a wealth of fitness information in a practical, fun and friendly way. This book will give you a good, basic fitness education.

The Rugged Walker by Patricia Kirk
Human Kinetics, Champaign, IL

> **Comments:** If you love exercising outdoors, you'll love this book. *The Rugged Walker* is a conditioning program for your body and your mind, which puts some fun and adventure into your exercise routine. If you like cruising, you'll also like rugged walking.

Too Busy To Exercise by Porter Shimer
Storey Publishing, Pownal, VT

> **Comments:** This book will help you find ways to fit exercise into your day. It is a concise fitness reference book for busy people and includes hundreds of useful tips.

4
A Half-Marathon
The Ultimate Confidence-Builder

> Vigorous exercise fills a man
> with pride and spirit, and he
> becomes twice the man he was.
>
> *Socrates*

Tom, an infrequent exerciser with a real desire to get in shape, came to me and wondered if I thought he would be able to join my Saturday cruising group. At six feet two inches tall and 250 pounds he certainly didn't look like the running type, but I told him he would be perfect for cruising and encouraged him to join the group.

Tom was somewhat intimidated at first since he feared he would be the slowest one in the group. He showed up every Saturday and became more motivated as he tacked on another mile and reached a new lifetime record each week. When he finally completed his first half-marathon, he was 15 pounds lighter and full of life. I cruised that race with him and all he kept saying was, "Why don't you go ahead of me so you can get a good time?" I had to remind him that cruising is not about getting the best time, it's about achieving your goals and having fun. I was having more fun talking with Tom and enjoying the beautiful scenery along the course.

We crossed the finish line together and Tom was thrilled with his accomplishment. He learned to believe in himself.

Cruise Your First Half-Marathon

How do you think you would feel after crossing the finish line of your first half-marathon, a 13.1 mile challenge? Fit? Proud? Confident? Definitely. Although it may seem like a big leap from the Base Training Program, achieving that goal is easier than you think.

Each year I look for a group of people who believe there is no way they could complete a half-marathon. I feel challenged to prove them wrong. So I convince them it is possible and guide them through my program. So far, every person who remained committed was successful and has gained more self-confidence.

If you completed the Base Training Program, you have grasped the concept of cruising and are in good condition to begin the 12-week Half-Marathon Program. A half-marathon is 13.1 miles; however, your training schedule still involves only three days a week of training. This program is designed to challenge you physically and mentally, and leave you feeling more confident than ever. Here are a few of the key components:

Weekday Workouts

The two weekday workouts are designed for heart and lungs conditioning. During these three-mile workouts, focus on improving your total time, even by a few seconds. These workouts should be challenging as they help to enhance fitness level and improve pace.

If you are able to run three miles without walking, do so during these weekday workouts. On the other hand, if you have identified a cruise plan that you enjoy and one that feels comfortable for your body, stick with it and cruise the three-mile workouts.

Weekend Workouts

The weekend workout is designed to condition your muscles, bones and joints and improve overall endurance. This workout teaches your body to use energy efficiently. Since this is the workout which increases in distance by about one mile each week, always cruise, even if you are able to run your weekday workouts without taking walking breaks. Keep in mind, during your weekend workout, going the distance is what is important, even if you do more walking than running.

For the weekend workout, unless you have identified your own personal cruise plan, try a 10:2 cruise plan. This workout is the essence of what cruising is all about, so be sure to keep it slow, easy and relaxed. Go at a pace that allows you to talk comfortably and enjoy your workout.

The Long Cruise

For this program, the long cruise is defined as one that is 10 miles or more. There are only two long cruises in the Half-Marathon program. Your weekend workout will get longer by one mile each week as you progress through the program. The long cruise helps to build endurance and strength. Remember to go slower during long cruises. Time is not important. Just go the distance. After every long cruise, it is important to give your body some rest by incorporating an easy week.

Easy Weeks

During a week marked "easy," forget about your total time and make your weekday workout easier. If you are running during those workouts, cruise instead. If you are already cruising, select an easier cruise plan. For example, if you are doing a 10:2 cruise, try a 5:1 cruise instead. Easy cruising weeks give your body some well-deserved rest and are designed for you to enjoy! During easy weeks, add more stretching after each workout (see Chapter 7). Most likely, after a week of easier exercise, you'll be stronger for your next workout.

Cruising Hills

If you have selected a half-marathon course that includes some hills, then it would be smart to incorporate some hill training into your workouts. Make one of your workouts a hill session during weeks 8 through 11. Hill training will make cruising your first half-marathon easier by strengthening your legs. In addition, because hill workouts are more intense, they burn more calories which is important if weight loss is one of your goals.

To enjoy workouts that include hills, be more flexible with your cruise plan. During your cruise, when you come upon a hill, slow down and walk briskly up it. Try to maintain an even breathing rate. As you near the crest of the hill, begin running again. To prevent injuries, be sure that when you are running down hills, you are light on your feet—run down hills relaxed and easy.

The Half-Marathon Cruising Program

	Day One (run or cruise)		Day Two (run or cruise)		Weekend (cruise 10:2)	
	MILES	TIME	MILES	TIME	MILES	TIME
Week 1	3		3		4	
Week 2	3		3		5	
Week 3	3		3		6	
Week 4 (easy)	3		3		7	
Week 5	3		3		8	
Week 6	3		3		9	
Week 7	3		3		10	
Week 8 (easy)	3		3		6 (hills)	
Week 9	3		3 (hills)		12	
Week 10 (easy)	3		3		6 (hills)	
Week 11	3		3 (hills)		6	
Week 12	3		3		13.1 Half-marathon	

A tracking chart is provided in the Appendix. After each cruise, record the total time it took you to complete the recommended distance.

Half Marathon Essentials

The essentials outlined in Chapter 2 are important for any cruising program; however, when training for a half-marathon, there are some additional thoughts to keep in mind.

Your Health. Training for a half-marathon is physically challenging. Be sure you have your physician's approval before starting this exercise program.

Your Goal. Even if your goal is to ultimately complete a marathon, be realistic. Set your half-marathon goal first and complete it. Some of my clients tried two or three half-marathons before training for a marathon.

The goal of this cruising program is to train you to finish your first half-marathon, so you cross the finish line feeling great, injury free, and having thoroughly enjoyed the experience. You will feel more self-confident and realize you can do just about anything in life you choose.

Your Schedule. Select a half-marathon and count back 12 weeks to determine your training start date. Choose the days for your weekday and weekend workouts. For half-marathon training, be sure to leave two full days of rest after your weekend workout. This gives your body a chance to recover after longer cruises.

Your Location. Since half-marathon training involves longer distances, it may take more work to find a place to train where you can add about one mile each week. If you want to include some hills, that too may take a bit of extra planning. Find a location that provides you the opportunity to refill your water bottle, use a rest-room or make a telephone call if necessary.

Your Running Shoes. To prevent excess wear, use your running shoes only for training. That is, don't wear them to the store or use them as "everyday" shoes. Once you have found a shoe that works great for you, stock up and buy a few pairs. (See Chapter 2 for more information about running shoes.)

Your Clothing. Experiment with clothing as your distances get longer. To prevent rashes from clothes rubbing, try flat-seamed apparel and avoid any clothing that is too tight. Running shorts are a good choice if your inner thighs don't rub and if you feel comfortable wearing them. Fabrics that wick moisture away from your skin are best, since they keep you cool when it's hot and keep you warm when it's cool. When training longer distances, you may want to consider wearing a neoprene runner's belt with pockets to hold energy bars, water, car keys, money, emergency medical information, sunscreen, sunglasses or anything else you want to have handy.

Your Partners. If you are exercising with a partner, as you complete longer distances, you each may progress at different rates. Your partner may have an easy day on one of your hard days. Be flexible, and if your goal is to stay together, be attentive to each others' needs. Don't push. Just tell yourselves to relax and enjoy.

Your Nutrition. As with any physical activity program, it is important that you eat well to stay fueled. Do not skip meals or try to exercise if you are feeling low on energy. When training longer distances, eat a light snack at least two hours before you exercise. Good nutrition is important to your success with this program (see Chapter 8).

Remember The Cruising Guidelines

The guidelines are presented in Chapter 2 and are so important, they are worth repeating. If you ever finish a workout and feel discouraged, ask yourself if you have followed the guidelines. Here they are again:

Cruising Guidelines

1. **Cruise three days a week; no more, no less.**

2. **Always warm up and cool down.**

3. **Use good form.**

4. **Take water breaks.**

5. **Be flexible.**

6. **Keep a positive attitude.**

Preparing For the Big Event

Race day is just around the corner. Assuming this is your first half-marathon, you need to be prepared. Knowing exactly what to do before, during and after the event can help contribute to your overall success. Review the following checklists to make sure you are prepared. You can also use these checklists anytime you are getting ready for a long cruise.

Preparation Checklists

Before the Race

- Stick with your training schedule. A general rule is to keep doing whatever you have been doing.

- Get at least two complete days of rest before the race.

- Clip your toenails.

- Drink plenty of water, especially a few days before the race (see Chapter 8).

- Relax and enjoy the company of family and friends.

- Plan to pack a bag for after the race which includes a fresh change of comfortable clothes, socks, water bottle, piece of fruit, energy bar or other snack.

- Gather your race instructions, bib and pins.

- Get a good night's sleep the night before the race.

Race Day

- Eat a light breakfast (see Chapter 8).

- Drink water. As a general guideline, drink 16 ounces up to two hours before the race and about four to eight ounces 5-10 minutes before.

- Get to the start line on time.

- This is not a must, but some experienced racers feel that it is a fashion "no-no" to wear your *finisher's* T-shirt on race day. You should wear it proudly *after* you finish.

During the Race

- Start out slowly! It is difficult to pace yourself when so many around you are passing you by. Let them pass. One of the biggest mistakes you can make is to start out too fast.

- Be flexible with your cruise plan. Perhaps you are using a 10:2 cruise plan and you come to a hill eight minutes into the race. Go ahead and walk up it. You may choose to take your walk breaks at every water station and when going up hills.

- Drink plenty of water, especially if the weather is hot. I recommend you carry a small water bottle. This way you can take frequent sips between water stations which helps to prevent that feeling of water sloshing around in your stomach.

The Finish Line

- Cross the finish line with pride and KEEP MOVING. You are not done!!! When in the finisher's chute, keep your legs moving by marching in place. Then quickly find an area where you can walk for *at least 10-20 minutes.*

- Grab some water and continue to sip it during your cool-down.

- Remember to stretch. Begin with your standing stretches, then find a grassy area where you can perform stretches in the seated and lying positions. Spend at least 10 minutes stretching (see Chapter 7).

- Only when you have finished your cool-down, will you be ready to find your family and friends. Take photos, enjoy the finish line snacks. You may also want to change into some dry clothes.

After The Race

- Take the next couple of days off to rest your body. Short walks are fine if you feel up to it. I usually recommend taking a day off from work to relax your body and mind.

- Eat healthy foods to replace the nutrients you may have lost during the event (see Chapter 8).

- Get quality sleep.

- Set a new goal right away. Many people experience "the blues" after the event and have difficulty getting motivated again. Do another half-marathon, 10K or other race. Continue training and try a marathon. Schedule time with your cruising partners and come up with some ongoing exercise plans.

You've Built Confidence! Now Keep It.

One day, I was out walking my dog with Stacie, my 15-year-old neighbor. Except for walking home from school every day and walking her dog regularly, she was definitely a non-exerciser. I asked her if she wanted to start training for a half-marathon and explained my cruising program. "Sure," she said, but I later found out that she only agreed because she didn't know me too well and wanted to be nice. She also told me she hated running because of how hard it was when she had to do it for P.E. class in school. I assured her that cruising is different and said I would prove it by training her.

We trained regularly and started out with the Base Training program. During her first few workouts, Stacie was skeptical and wondered how she would ever be able to complete 13.1 miles. She stuck with it (to be nice) and each week became more confident as she tacked on one more mile.

Twelve weeks later, Stacie found herself cruising her first half-marathon. I waited for her at the finish line to place the finisher's medal around her neck. After achieving her goal, she said "It's all over. What now?"

Keep Cruising!

After completing the Half-Marathon Program, you have several options to keep yourself exercising. What you choose may be influenced by your experience with the half-marathon.

- Stay with the goal of cruising three times a week and make your weekend workout longer or cruise 10 miles once every month.

- Try the Marathon Cruising Program (Stacie was so motivated from the half-marathon, she went on to run two marathons in her first year of training!)

- Set a goal of completing one or two half-marathons each year and try different races and locations (see *The Largest Half-Marathons and Other Moderate Distance Races* at the end of this chapter).

- Enjoy your accomplishment and stay motivated by entering 5K and 10K road races a few times each year.

If you are interested in pursuing other fitness activities, review the Recommended Resources at the end of Chapters 3, 5 and 6. Just make a commitment to keep going!

The Largest Half-Marathons and Other Moderate-Distance Races in the U.S.

The following races are between seven miles and a half-marathon. Keep in mind, large races, where there are lots of runners and spectators, help keep you motivated.

Race	Location	Month
Lilac Bloomsday Run 12K (7.4 miles)	Spokane, WA	May
Bay to Breakers 12K (7.4 miles)	San Francisco, CA	May
Great Aloha Run 8.25 miles	Honolulu, HI	February
Quad-City Times Bix 7 7 miles	Davenport, IA	July
Indianapolis Life 500 13.1 miles	**Indianapolis, IN**	**May**
Army 10-Miler 10 miles	Washington, DC	October
Falmouth Road Race 7.1 miles	Falmouth, MA	August
Philadelphia Distance Run – 13.1 miles	**Philadelphia, PA**	**September**
Gate River Run 15K (9.3 miles)	Jacksonville, FL	March
Sound to Narrows 12K (7.4 miles)	Tacoma, WA	June
Atlanta Half-Marathon 13.1 miles	**Atlanta, GA**	**November**

Race	Location	Month
Utica Boilermaker 15K (9.3 miles)	Utica, NY	July
Gasparilla Distance 15K (9.3 miles)	Tampa, FL	January
Dallas YMCA Turkey Trot – 8 miles	Dallas, TX	November
Nortel Cherry Blossom 10 miles	Washington, DC	April
Crim Festival of Races 10 miles	Flilnt, MI	August
America's Finest City 13.1 miles	**San Diego, CA**	**August**
Broad Street Run 10 miles	Philadelphia, PA	May
Kentucky Derby Festival – 13.1 miles	**Louisville, KY**	**April**

5
Your First Marathon
You Can Do It, If You Cruise It

> A man's reach should exceed his grasp.
>
> *Robert Browning*

Peggy is a huge Oprah fan and was so inspired when Oprah ran a marathon for her 40th birthday, she began telling her friends and family that she wanted to do the same. Peggy, who casually ran short distances for a good part of her life, tried training for the City of Los Angeles Marathon by joining a local running group. She made it up to 11 miles, but then had to drop out because of a serious knee injury. To heal, she had to stop running.

Every time Peggy tried to run again, after about a month of running, four to five days a week, her knee became swollen and painful. As her 40th birthday approached, she knew she only had one more year to give it a try. She asked for my help and I recommended the cruising program. Peggy explained her knee problem and her fear of being injured again.

After getting the "thumbs-up" from her doctor, she began the cruising program. I explained that with this program she would have to cut back her running to two days a week plus the weekend workout, which she would be cruising. At first she was reluctant because she wanted to lose some weight and thought that running every day was the answer. "Moderation is the key," I said and with cruising there is a strong emphasis on preventing injury. I recommended she do low-impact activities such as walking, biking or swimming on her "off" days.

Peggy continued with the cruising program and was able to talk her boyfriend into joining her (he agreed to try it, but only up to ten miles). She added some cycling and weight training because she felt the cruising program was easy for her. Before she knew it, she was up to 13 miles, a distance she had never before been able to reach.

After successfully completing a half-marathon, Peggy knew she was on her way. Not only had she lost 18 pounds by simply cutting back, something she had been trying to do for the past 20 years, but her knees felt great. She looked and felt fit. "Just a few more long cruises and you're ready for the marathon," I told her.

Peggy made it! She crossed the Los Angeles Marathon finish line a new woman. Fit and forty! No injuries. No problems. "Life really does begin at 40, she said" Oprah knows it. Now Peggy knows it too.

You Can Do It!

Once you complete your first marathon, you'll understand why millions of people do it each year. It's not about running or fitness. It's about accomplishment and it involves believing in yourself. It teaches you a lot about life. I remember when I cruised my first marathon, I found it interesting to read the backs of runners' T-shirts as I slowly passed them by. Here is a sample of what I read:

"This time last year I was a heroin addict"
"I'm 72 and proud of it!"
"I can do anything, if I can do this"
"In loving memory of my dad"

Some T-shirts actually brought tears to my eyes. I could relate to some of the reasons why people were running the marathon. I was close to someone struggling with a drug problem. My dad passed away that year. My mom was approaching 70. This incredible physical challenge is also a powerful, positive force that can change lives.

Don't let anyone tell you that you are crazy for wanting to try a marathon. It is an unbelievable experience that not many people attempt. You could consider yourself among a very select, special group of individuals. I know you can do it because every person that I have trained since I developed this program has succeeded. Most, started out as non-exercisers or runners with history of injury. The most important thing for you to know is that the cruising program makes it possible by keeping the training moderate and easy on your body. What is even more amazing is watching your body transform. I won't lie and tell you that it won't be physically and mentally challenging at times, but you will love the results!

Cruise Your First Marathon

The Marathon Cruising Program is 24 weeks. It's identical to the Half-Marathon Program up to the middle of Week 12, so if you just completed that training, you can keep going and start the marathon program at Week 11 to allow yourself enough recovery from the half-marathon. The program is moderate and designed to help you succeed. Here is a reminder about the key components of the Marathon Program.

Weekday Workouts

Unlike many traditional marathon training programs, these workouts don't change. They are still three miles and able to fit nicely into a busy schedule. Continue to focus on improving your total time.

Weekend Workouts

Similar to the half-marathon training weekend workout, this will increase in distance after 10 miles, but only every two or three weeks. When training beyond 10-12 miles, allow yourself a longer cool-down. Most of my clients chose to walk the last mile or two and noticed a dramatic decrease in muscle soreness. Remember to keep this cruise slow, easy and relaxed.

Try a 10:2 cruise plan. This helps train your body to walk about every mile or so, depending on your pace. In a marathon, this works great because you end up walking at most of the water stations. Some of my clients have used a 20:3 cruise plan for marathons. The 20:3 cruising plan worked especially well for those people who preferred to maintain an even rhythm for a longer period of time. You can experiment with different cruise plans during the training program to find what works best for you.

The Long Cruise

In Week 15, 18 and 21 you have your longest cruises. Cruise the distance and finish by walking 2 miles. For example, in Week 15 the distance goal is 16-18 miles. This means you cruise up to 16 and walk for two miles, covering a total distance of 18 miles. This helps reduce soreness and speeds recovery from the long cruise. DO NOT neglect to do the two miles of walking, even if you feel up to continuing your cruise plan. The extra walking makes an incredible difference in how you will feel the next day.

Easy Weeks

After any long cruise, enjoy a week of easier exercise and you'll come back stronger. Your body needs and deserves some rest. During easy weeks you should do shorter distances and take more frequent walking breaks. Keep in mind, easy weeks help you recover from your long cruises.

Cruising Hills

Make one of your workouts each week a hill session during Weeks 11 through 20. Whether you choose to run or walk up the hills, this type of training will help make your first marathon easier.

The Marathon Cruising Program

	Day One (run or cruise)		Day Two (run or cruise)		Weekend (cruise 10:2 or 20:3)	
	MILES	TIME	MILES	TIME	MILES	TIME
Week 1	3		3		4	
Week 2	3		3		5	
Week 3	3		3		6	
Week 4	3		3		7	
Week 5	3		3		8	
Week 6	3		3		9	
Week 7	3		3		10	
Week 8	3		3		6	
Week 9	3		3		12	
Week 10	3		3		6	
Week 11	3		3		6 hills	
Week 12	3 hills		3		14	
Week 13	2-3		2-3		6 hills	
Week 14	3		3		6 hills	
Week 15	3 hills		3		16-18	
Week 16	2-3		2-3		6 hills	
Week 17	3		3		6 hills	
Week 18	3 hills		3		18-20	
Week 19	2-3		2-3		6 hills	
Week 20	3		3		6 hills	
Week 21	3		3		20-22	
Week 22	2-3		2-3		6	
Week 23	3		3		6	
Week 24	3		3		26.2	

Marathon Essentials

The cruising essentials outlined in Chapter 2 and expanded in Chapter 4 are important. Review them again before training for a full marathon and keep these additional thoughts in mind:

Your Health. Once you have your physician's approval to train for a marathon, be sure to keep yourself in good health during your training. Do not try to continue training if you become ill or injured. Simply back off for a while and give your body a chance to heal. You can always continue your training when feeling better.

Your Goal. Keep in mind, the goal here is simply *to finish* your first marathon. Time is not important; feeling great about your accomplishment is.

Your Schedule. Select a marathon and count back 24 weeks to determine your training start date or continue your half-marathon training by starting the Marathon Cruising Program at Week 11. Send in your marathon entry form once you've completed the 16-18 mile training cruise. This will help keep you motivated and strengthen your commitment. You are almost there.

Your Nutrition. During this program, it is important to keep your body well-nourished, especially before the long cruises. You must drink plenty of water and may even need to eat a light snack during your longer exercise sessions. (See Chapter 8 for more information.)

Remember The Cruising Guidelines

Follow the Cruising Guidelines presented in Chapter 2. If necessary, review them again and again. They hold the key to your success.

Cruising Guidelines

1. **Cruise three days a week; no more, no less.**

2. **Always warm up and cool down.**

3. **Use good form.**

4. **Take water breaks.**

5. **Be flexible.**

6. **Keep a positive attitude.**

The Big Event -26.2

Review the checklists in Chapter 4 and the nutrition information in Chapter 8 to be sure you know exactly how to prepare for the marathon. These preparation checklists are helpful when getting ready for any long-distance workout, including those that are part of your training.

Since finishing a marathon is a tremendous physical and mental challenge, I suggest placing just as much importance on your recovery as you did for your training. Below is a marathon recovery program I developed based on client feedback as well as my own experiences.

After The Race - Recovery Week

Once again, this is the most important part of the program. You will need to spend the entire week after the marathon focusing on your health. This week is a time when your body's resistance is low and you are more prone to catching a cold, flu or other infection. Even if you feel great, take the time to focus on recovery.

- Take at least one day off from work to relax your body and mind. Schedule a massage, get a pedicure and take a Yoga or other stretching-type class. Short walks are fine during the first two recovery days, if you feel up to it. Just be sure to keep the walks slow and easy.

- Take care of any injuries. Use ice, even for the slightest aches and pains, regularly for one week. When icing a body part, use an ice pack that has a cover or put a thin cloth between the ice pack and your skin to prevent frostbite. Ice only for 10-15 minutes a couple times during the day. This should help reduce any inflammation and speed recovery.

- Stretch at least 15 minutes every day (see Chapter 7).

- Eat healthy foods to replace the nutrients you may have lost during the event. Focus on foods such as fresh fruits and juices, vegetables, pasta, grains and cereals. Go out for dinner and order your favorite meal, complete with salad and dessert. Instead of focusing on eating low fat, try to make all your food choices ones that are packed with nutrients. Good nutrition will help speed the recovery process.

- Get quality sleep for the entire week. If possible, try to wake up without the use of an alarm. Wash your sheets and pillows to make your bed as comfortable as possible.

- Take extra care to manage your level of stress. Try taking a warm bath everyday. Set out some candles around the bathtub, get a good book and just relax.

- Think about setting a new goal. Schedule time with your cruising partners and come up with some ongoing exercise plans. Below is a four-week marathon recovery exercise program that keeps you moving three days a week. Use this program to keep you motivated while you are setting a new goal. At the end of the program you should be able to resume your normal cruising schedule.

Marathon Recovery for Cruisers

Week 1

Three days after the marathon, walk 2-3 miles at a comfortable pace. During the week, add one more day of comfortable walking. On the weekend after the marathon, walk 2-3 miles or perform 30 minutes of a different activity, such as swimming, bicycling, roller-skating or other low to moderate-intensity exercise.

Week 2

Cruise 2-3 miles twice during the week and once on the weekend. For these workouts, use a 5:3 cruise plan. If you prefer performing 30 minutes of a different activity instead of a cruise, do so on the weekends. This can give your body and mind a rest from your usual workouts.

Week 3

Cruise three miles twice during the week and once on the weekend. For these workouts, use a 10:3 cruise plan.

| Week 4 | Cruise three miles twice during the week and once on the weekend. For these workouts, use any cruise plan you feel comfortable with or run all |

three miles. By the end of Week 4, you should feel fully recovered.

Enjoy Your Achievement!

Just after my first marathon in 1994, I invited my cruising partners, friends and family to my house for a post-race barbecue. It was time to celebrate. We proudly wore our finisher T-shirts and medals the rest of the day. I also invited a new acquaintance, Donny, who later became my husband. That following year, I trained him for his first marathon.

The 1995 Los Angeles Marathon, was my most memorable. Not just because I was cruising with Donny, celebrating the one year anniversary of our first date, but because it rained—heavily. We woke up that morning, looked outside and he said, "Now what do we do coach?" Well, once you have trained six months for your first marathon, it seems like it would be a waste NOT to do it. Donny and I decided to dress for cruising in the rain, which meant sticking your head and arms through a large plastic garbage bag (that's what all the other runners were doing). The gun went off and we went splashing along with 20,000 others while the Los Angeles Marathon theme song, "I Love L.A." (rain or shine), played to start us on our way.

There is a certain energy present at large marathons, especially when it's raining. It's like everyone has taken the "nothing will stop me" attitude. It's amazing to see how many people refuse to use the weather as an excuse to give up. Despite the pounding rain and strong winds, Donny and I made our way along the course. At about the halfway mark we thought about calling it quits. It was raining so hard, we could barely see. It was a good thing I stuffed a $20 bill in my shorts, because we decided to cruise into a shoe store on Hollywood Boulevard and buy some dry socks. I handed the clerk my soggy $20 bill and once again, we were on our way to the finish line.

There were times when we thought the rain would stop, but it didn't. Being from the East Coast, all I kept thinking about was how big the rain drops are in California and how fast the streets become flooded. At times we were in puddles up to our ankles. It made us feel slow and heavy. We wondered how many extra pounds of water we were dragging along.

At about mile 19 it became a mental challenge. I didn't want to finish. Donny did and reminded me where we were — only seven miles from the finish line. He pointed to all the spectators who came out with umbrellas to cheer us on and said, "This is the beautiful part of Los Angeles — the people." He was right. There were still bands playing music and people dancing in the rain. Although physically it was the toughest, it was also the most inspiring part of the marathon. How amazing it was to see such support from the spectators. There were children holding their hands out in hopes of getting a "high-five" from a runner. It was at this moment I discovered that completing a marathon is not about running, but about people coming together and about life. Nothing could stop us now.

We splashed across the finish line together and the celebration continued. The party has never ended. Each year I look forward to inspiring just one more person who believes completing a marathon is impossible.

Once you complete your first marathon, you will be an inspiration to others. You may even change someone else's life. You will realize that just about anything in life is possible. So once you do this, savor every moment after you cross the finish line. Take pictures, have a party, frame your medal, talk about it with friends and family. Enjoy your achievement.

Keep Cruising

What next? Can anything top the high you feel after completing your first marathon? Hurry. Set another goal quick before the post-marathon blues set in. Almost everyone feels a bit sad when it's all over and during the recovery period, you may begin to lose motivation to exercise. Recover fully, then spend some time deciding on a new goal. You could always go back to cruising or running three times a week, but if you don't have a specific goal in mind, you may lose interest. Here are some options to keep yourself motivated:

- Register for a shorter distance race within the next month.

- Commit to doing one marathon per year and try to improve your time each year.

- Use the off-season to focus on strength training and stretching.

- Pick up some running books to find out how to take your training to the next level (see Recommended Resources at the end of this chapter).

- Look into other outdoor fitness activities such as biking, hiking or roller-skating.

- Keep cruising or running three days a week, trying to improve your speed.

- Get one other person involved in this program and see that person through his or her accomplishment. You will get a tremendous sense of satisfaction from inspiring others. Give *Just Cruising* as a gift to someone you would like to train with and as a nonmaterial gift, you can be that person's partner and mentor.

Recommended Resources

Marathon Training: The Proven 100-Day Program for Success by Joe Henderson
Human Kinetics, Champaign, IL

> **Comments:** This book includes all the key information about marathon training and guides you through a 15-week program, day-by-day with information, tips and a training log. Henderson even has a program for cruisers!

Marathon by Jeff Galloway
Phiddipides Publications, Atlanta, GA

> **Comments:** This books focuses on the marathon. So if you want to do another marathon, check out this book. It includes training programs for specific time goals. For all you cruisers, there is an excellent chapter on the value of walking breaks. See if you can make someone else a believer.

Healthy Runner's Handbook by Lyle J. Micheli
Human Kinetics, Champaign, IL

> **Comments:** This is a good resource for injuries and prevention. The 31 most common injuries are addressed. This is not to say you will become injured, but more importantly, you will learn about how to prevent injuries and care for one, should it happen.

The Essential Marathoner by John Hanc
Lyons & Buford Publishers, New York, NY

> **Comments:** This book is a concise guide to training
> for the marathon. It provides an easy training schedule
> and gives sound advice. It is much smaller than the
> above references, so if you want to read something
> quick and easy, this is it.

6
Getting Strong
Simple, At-Home Workouts for Cruisers

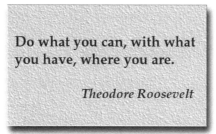

Do what you can, with what you are.

Theodore Roosevelt

Strength training, also known as resistance exercise, toning and muscle conditioning, is an essential part of a well-rounded fitness program. This type of exercise provides resistance to muscles, making them stronger over time. There are many benefits of having a strong body:

- Strong muscles help make cruising and other daily physical activities easier.

- Improved muscular strength helps prevent injuries by helping to protect joints.

- Stronger muscles burn more calories which is important for weight loss and weight maintenance.

- Strength training helps build bone density which may reduce your risk of osteoporosis (bone disease) and is especially important for women over 50.

- Increased strength of the torso and postural muscles helps reduce your risk of back problems.

- A stronger, more muscular and toned body may help you look and feel better.

Improvements in muscular strength can occur at all ages, so it's never too late to start a strength training program. There are many simple exercises that can be done in your own home, without exercise equipment.

Strengthen Your Cruise

If you are the type of person who prefers unstructured exercise, here are some strength training ideas you can incorporate into your everyday activities.

Walk Hills

If you like walking or hiking, find some hills. Walking up steep hills, forward *and* backward, does wonders for strengthening your legs. Since cruising strengthens mainly the back of the legs and hips, walking backward up hills is especially good for improving strength in the front of your legs, thereby promoting a better balance of strength.

Stand on One Foot

Pick up one foot at least an inch off the floor by slightly bending the knee of the leg you are lifting. Stand up straight for a minute or two, then switch to the other leg. This is a great exercise for strengthening your ankles and hips. It also helps to improve your balance.

Sit Upright

When sitting at work or at home, think about your posture. Be sure you are sitting erect with your shoulders back and chest forward. The next time you are watching television or talking on the phone, sit perfectly erect for five minutes. You will be amazed at how tired your upper back muscles become. The harder it is for you to sit up straight, the more you need postural exercises. As you become stronger, gradually increase the amount of time for this exercise. Not only will strong postural muscles help prevent back problems, but it will make you look and feel more confident.

Toe Taps

Take a few minutes during your day to tap your feet, as if tapping to the beat of music. It will help you improve strength in your shin muscles. This is an important exercise for cruisers since walking and running emphasizes use of the calf muscles (in the back of your lower legs) which can sometimes lead to a muscle imbalance (strong calves, but weak shin muscles) and injury.

Keep Tight Abs

The abdominal muscles function to hold our bodies in an upright position and help to maintain proper posture. A simple abdominal exercise you can do involves tightening your abdominal muscles. Hold the position for five to 10 seconds and relax. This exercise can be performed in the sitting or standing position and can be held for longer periods of time.

Getting Equipped

If you are willing to make a small investment in some equipment items, you will have a much wider variety of exercise options available. This can help to keep your strength workouts challenging which may also help you to stay motivated. The equipment recommended here is inexpensive and can meet a variety of needs. Your local sporting goods store should carry most of these items or you can refer to the mail-order sources listed at the end of this chapter.

Wrist/Ankle Weights

There are a variety of exercises that can be done using wrist/ankle weights. Get the adjustable and washable type if possible. A 5-pound pair is sufficient; however, a heavier pair will accommodate increases in strength. The heavier weights are more expensive. Wrist/ankle weights are for strength development only and should not be worn during cruising workouts.

Dumbbells

You can work just about every major muscle group with dumbbells. To save money and space, look for the adjustable type. This way, as you get stronger, you can gradually add more weight without going out and purchasing more dumbbells.

Exercise Ball

The large air-filled vinyl ball, also known as a Swiss ball, offers some excellent exercise choices. The ball challenges your balance so you work many muscles at the same time, thus speeding up your workout. It is most effective for strengthening the abdominal and back muscles, but you can exercise nearly every muscle group with the ball. The ball also allows you to exercise in positions unattainable on the floor or on other pieces of equipment. Often, these positions are safer and more comfortable for your body.

> Be sure the ball is correctly sized for your body. Knees and hips should be bent at 90 degree angles when sitting upright on the ball. A 55 cm ball is generally recommended for adults between 5 and 6 feet and a 65 cm ball for those over 6 feet. You can vary the size by inflating or deflating the ball slightly.

Tubing/Bands

There are several types of elastic resistance products and many ways to use them. For the exercises presented in this book, I recommend tubing with handles. Purchase two light-resistance and two medium-resistance tubes. As you become stronger, you will need to increase the resistance. Start by doubling up on the light resistance, then try a medium and a light and then two or three mediums. Tubing is excellent to take along when traveling because it's light and compact. Store tubing and bands away from heat and sunlight.

Create Your Own Strength Workout

When it comes to strength, everyone has different needs, interests and abilities. Some people also have physical limitations. Put together your own workout by selecting one exercise from each group presented in this chapter until you have a total of 10 exercises. Change your workout every six to eight weeks to keep your body challenged and your mind interested. If you invest in some of the recommended equipment items, you will have a wider variety of exercise options.

Follow The Strength Guidelines

The strength guidelines here are designed to help improve strength and muscular endurance. Muscular endurance is the ability of a muscle to work against resistance many times; therefore, you will notice the guidelines call for higher repetitions of each exercise than standard guidelines for muscular strength. This type of training is more specific to cruising, yet offers the same benefits: muscle strength and tone.

1. Perform your strength workout a minimum of two days a week.

This is realistic for busy people. Spread the days out over the entire week, and if you choose days you are not cruising, each day's workout will be no longer than 30 minutes. For example, if you are cruising Tuesday, Thursday and Saturday, you may want to do your strength workout on Mondays and Fridays or Sundays and Wednesdays. If you are consistent for at least three weeks and have the extra time, you may want to add another day of strength training. You will see faster results, but it is more difficult to stick to a three-day strength schedule. You may also alternate, three days one week, then two days the next and so on. Just be sure to leave at least 48 hours between strength workouts which gives your muscles a chance to recover and become stronger.

2. Always warm up.

Start your strength training workout with three to five minutes of walking or jogging in place to prepare your muscles. Then perform some brief stretching exercises for each body part (see Chapter 7).

3. Start with one set of 15-18 repetitions of each exercise.

This high-repetition recommendation is more appropriate for cruisers, or endurance exercisers, who want to improve muscular endurance and tone. Progress to two sets after three weeks if your time allows. When doing two sets, allow about one to one and a half minutes between each set.

4. Use a resistance that allows you to do at least 15 reps, but no more than 18.

If your muscles are not tired by 18 repetitions, then the resistance may be too light. If you have difficulty reaching 15 repetitions, keep at it and work your way up or lower the resistance. It is always better to be conservative when evaluating the resistance. Before increasing resistance, perform each exercise two seconds slower for the next three workouts. If the exercise is still too easy, then it is time to increase the resistance.

5. Perform each repetition slowly.

As a general rule, take six seconds per repetition. This translates to three seconds for each lifting movement (or execution of the exercise) and three seconds for the lowering movement (or return to starting position).

6. Use proper technique.

Look at each exercise photo carefully and copy the technique. Read the cues for each photo. If possible, use a mirror to check your form.

About The Exercises

It is important to get a balanced muscular workout by exercising opposing muscle groups. For example, if you choose a chest exercise, you should also choose an upper back exercise. The exercises that follow are grouped according to major muscle groups. Choose one exercise from each group and you will end up with a balanced workout consisting of ten exercises. The workout should take about 20-25 minutes to complete.

I have selected the exercises that are safest for your joints and most effective for a wide variety of individuals. These exercises are also specific to helping improve your cruising performance. Copy and enlarge the chart at the end of this chapter and use it to record your workouts.

A Word About Muscular Imbalance

Most strength experts agree that all major muscle groups should be exercised in a strength training program; however, running can cause tight, overdeveloped rear leg muscles (gluteals, hamstrings and calves), while doing little for the front leg muscles (quadriceps and shins). Therefore, some individuals who choose mostly running while cruising may end up with an imbalance in the strength ratio between the front and rear leg muscles. Muscle "imbalance" can lead to injuries. For this reason, many running experts recommend a focus on **strengthening the front leg muscles** and **stretching the rear leg muscles**.

While a muscular imbalance is uncommon for short-distance cruisers, it can occur with regular, long-distance training. If you suspect you have a muscle imbalance in your legs (chronic injuries or tightness that does not go away with stretching and rest), seek the advice of a physical therapist or sports physician who can evaluate your leg strength and recommend the appropriate exercises.

Group 1 - QUADRICEPS (front of thigh)

OPEN SQUAT

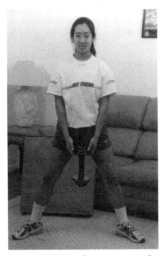

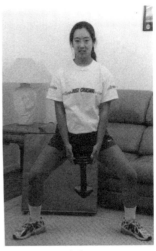

1-1A Turn feet outward. Keep back straight.

1-1B Bend knees; return to start. Keep knees over centers of feet.

SIDE STEP-UP

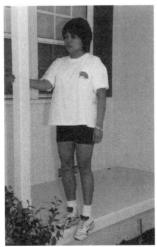

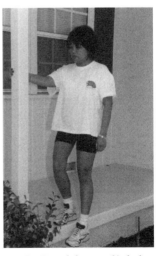

1-2A Use 4-6" step or curb. Hold railing for balance.

1-2B Bend knee slightly; return to start. Keep weight on back 2/3 of supporting foot. Keep back straight.

STANDING LEG EXTENSION
(with tubing or band)

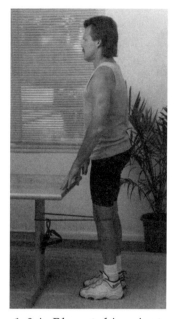

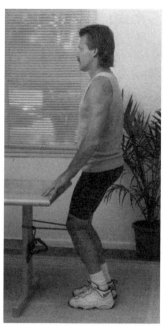

1-3B Bend knee slightly; return to start. Keep heels on floor and back straight.

1-3A Place tubing just above knee. Tie to sturdy object. Keep back straight.

Neutral Spine

For most exercises, keep your spine in a neutral (or its natural) position. This means your lower back should not be excessively arched nor your upper back rounded. Keep good posture at all times during exercise; even when cruising.

BALL SQUAT

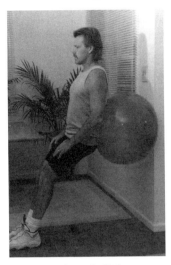

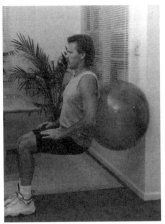

1-4A Place ball between wall and lower back. Keep back straight and upright. Legs should have slight bend in knees.

1-4B Bend knees until in a seated position with knees at a 90 degree angle; press back up to start. Hold weights for more resistance. (This exercise may also be done just sliding against a smooth wall.)

STRAIGHT LEG LIFT

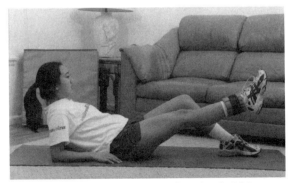

1-5 Keep back straight with spine held in a neutral position. Lift and lower leg. Use an ankle weight for more resistance.

Group 2 - HAMSTRINGS (back of thigh)

CHAIR SQUAT

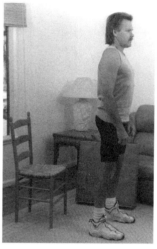

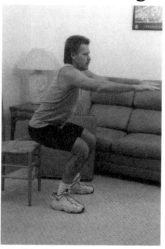

2-1A Stand with feet hip-width apart and position chair behind you.

2-1B Squat as if preparing to sit while reaching arms forward; return to start. Keep back straight and weight on back 2/3 of feet.

LEG CURL

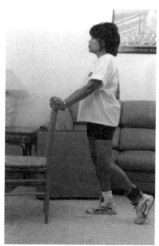

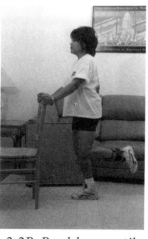

2-2A Hold chair or counter for balance.

2-2B Bend knee until lower leg is parallel to floor; return to start. Keep knees aligned.

SEATED LEG CURL

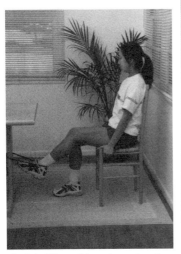

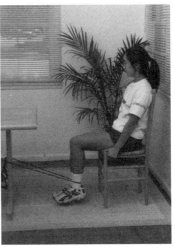

2-3A Tie tubing to a sturdy object and place around ankle. Sit with back straight.

2-3B Bend knee, bringing ankle toward chair; return to start. Keep working leg slightly lifted.

BALL LEG CURL

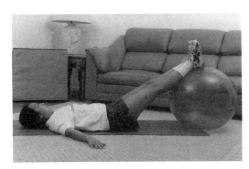

2-4A Place heels on center of ball. Angle arms out to sides for balance.

2-4B Bend knees and roll ball inward while pressing heels into ball. Lift back off floor for more challenge. Keep a neutral spine.

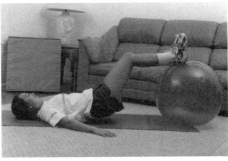

Group 3 - SHINS (front of lower leg)

SEATED TOE LIFT

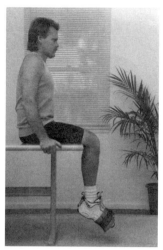

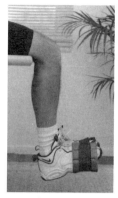

3-1B Lift toes upward as high as possible; return to start.

3-1A Sit erect on table or counter. Place weights around tops of feet with toes pointing downward.

STANDING TOE LIFT

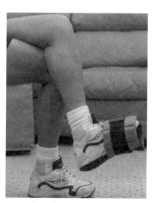

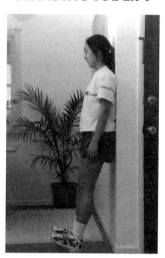

3-1C This exercise may also be done seated in a chair, one leg at a time.

3-2 Stand with feet 10-12" from wall, keeping back straight and against wall. Lift toes upward; return to start.

Group 4 - CALVES (back of lower leg)

CALF RAISE

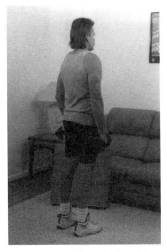

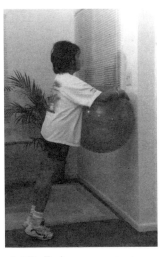

4-1A Stand with feet hip-width apart and parallel.

4-1B Raise up onto toes; return to start. Lean against a wall for help with balance.

BALL CALF RAISE

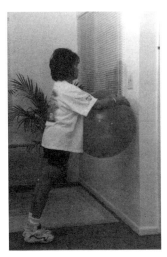

4-2A Lean body on a slight angle against ball.

4-2B Raise up onto toes, pressing body against ball; return to start.

Group 5 - CHEST & FRONT OF SHOULDERS

COUNTER PUSH-UP

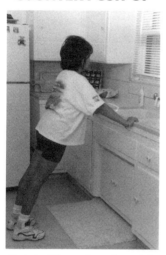

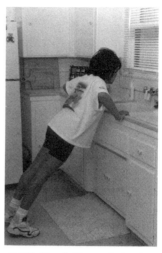

5-1A Place hands wide apart on a dry counter.

5-1B Bend elbows, bringing chest to edge of counter; return to start. Keep body straight.

About Hand Position for Push-ups

Place hands wide enough apart so that when elbows are in the bent position, there is a 90 degree angle at the elbow joint. Angle hands slightly inward. Lower body only as far as you can control.

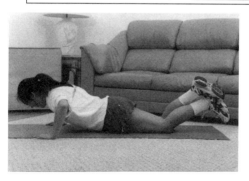

PUSH-UP

5-2 May be done on floor with bent knees. From head to knees, keep body straight.

FULL PUSH-UP

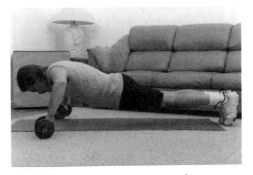

5-3 To ease pressure on wrists, use dumbbells to keep wrists extended. From head to heels, keep body straight.

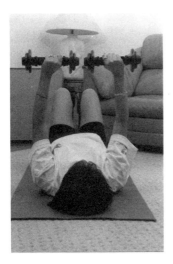

CHEST PRESS

5-4A   Hold ends of dumbbells together, centered over chest. Keep shoulder blades pressed against floor to stabilize upper back.

5-4B   Bend elbows and lower weight until elbows are bent 90 degrees. Stop before elbows touch floor; return to start.

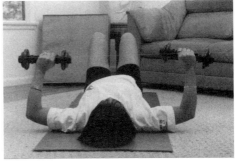

Group 6 - UPPER BACK & BACK OF SHOULDERS

SEATED ROW

6-1A Wrap tubing around feet. Sit with back straight, knees slightly bent and palms facing inward.

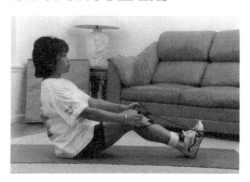

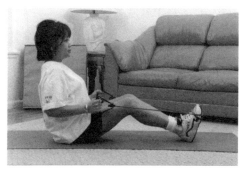

6-1B Bend elbows, and pull back while squeezing shoulder blades together. Keep forearms parallel to the floor; return to start.

STANDING ROW

Upper Back Tip

When performing back exercises, start by squeezing the shoulder blades together to engage the postural muscles.

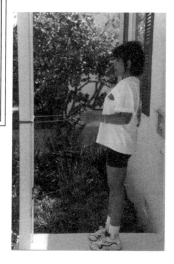

6-2 This exercise may also be done in a standing position. Wrap tubing around a fence, post or railing.

DUMBBELL PULLOVER

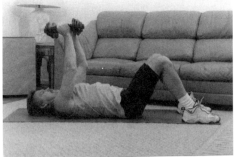

6-3A Hold weight centered over chest. Keep elbows straight or just slightly bent.

6-3B Extend arms over head, stopping when upper arms are near face; return to start.

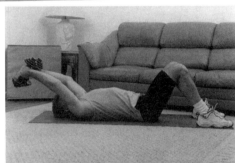

PULLDOWN
(with tubing)

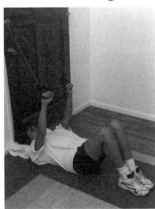

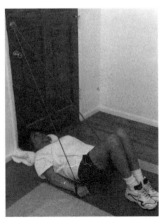

6-4A Loop tubing around secure object (i.e., door lock, door knob, railing).

6-4B Keeping elbows and wrists straight, pull fists downward to floor; return to start. Maintain a neutral spine.

Group 7 - BICEPS (front of upper arm)

ARM CURL

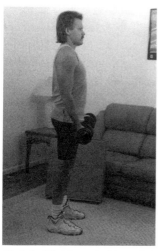

7-1A Hold weight, with palms facing forward.

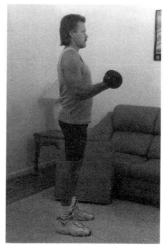

7-1B Bend elbows, lifting weight toward chest; return to start. Keep back and wrists straight and elbows near waist.

ARM CURL
(with tubing)

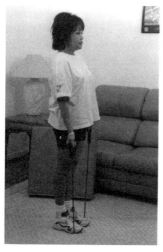

7-2A Place tubing under feet, close to toes.

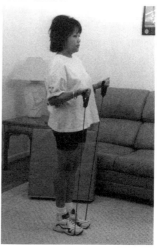

7-2B Pull upward without moving elbows away from waist; return to start. Keep wrists straight.

Group 8 - TRICEPS (back of upper arm)

PRESSDOWN
(with tubing)

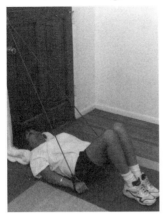

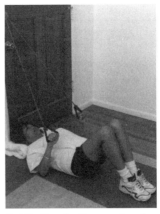

8-1B Bend elbows slowly, as far as possible with control; return to start. Keep upper arms on floor and close to body.

8-1A Loop tubing around secure object (i.e., door lock, door knob, railing). Pull fists downward to floor (see 6-4A&B).

TRICEPS PRESS

8-2A Keep arm vertical and wrist straight. Press shoulder blade to floor.

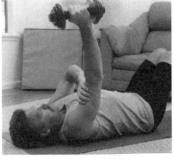

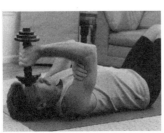

8-2B Bend elbow as far as possible with control; return to start. Keep upper arm vertical at all times.

Group 9 - ABDOMINALS AND WAIST

AB CRUNCH

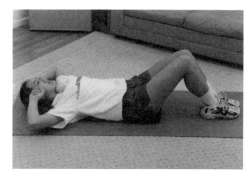

9-1A Place fists on temples. To maintain neutral neck position, place small ball under chin.

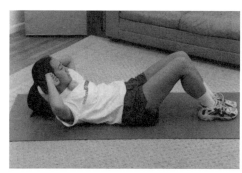

9-1B Lift by bringing rib cage toward hip bones; return to start.

9-2 To work the waist, add a twist while lifting. Keep back and hips on the floor.

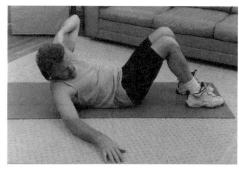

PRESS AND REACH

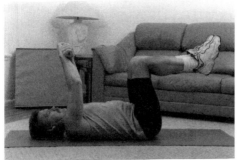

9-3A Start with arms crossed at wrists and hips and knees at 90 degree angles. Press back to floor.

9-3B Extend arms over head and one leg out. Keep back pressed to floor by tightening abdominal muscles.

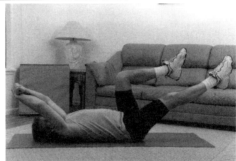

BALL CRUNCH

9-4A Center ball under low back and keep hips slightly lower than rib cage. Place fists at temples or arms across chest (easier).

9-4B Curl your trunk, bringing rib cage toward hips, allowing upper back to come off ball; return to start.

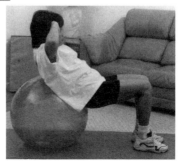

Group 10 - LOW BACK

OPPOSITE ARM/LEG LIFT

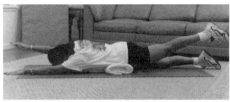

10-1 Lift one arm and opposite leg; pause, repeat on other side.

10-2 Use the ball for more challenge.

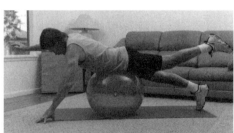

BACK EXTENSION ON BALL

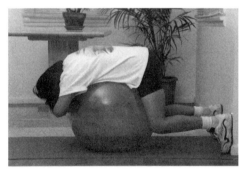

10-3A Round body over ball. Fold arms and place head against forearms. Brace feet against wall (if needed).

10-3B Extend to a neutral spine position; return to start. Keep head in contact with arms.

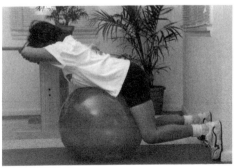

Keep It Simple and Be Strong

Keep your workout simple and change it often. If you are interested in learning more about strength training or ordering some home equipment products, check out the following resources:

Weight Training for Dummies by Liz Neporent and Suzanne Schlosberg—IDG Books Worldwide, Foster City, CA

> **Comments:** This book is an excellent guide for those who want to learn more about strength training. It is written for the beginner and includes information about home exercise equipment, weight training etiquette, how to choose a personal trainer, exercising in a health club and how to design a program. There is a helpful chapter on weight training jargon, which is essential for anyone new to exercise.

SPRI Products, Inc., 1026 Campus Drive, Mundelein, IL 60060—(800) 222-7774 or in Illinois call (847) 680-7774
www.fitnessonline.com

> **Comments:** Call for a fitness products catalog. This company sells elastic tubing/bands, exercise balls, dumbbells, ankle weights and more. They also have videos, exercise guidebooks, sport-specific training programs and fitness products for children.

Fitness Wholesale, 895-A Hampshire Road, Stow, OH 44224-1121—(800) 537-5512
www.fitnesswholesale.com

> **Comments:** Call for a fitness products catalog. This company also sells various small equipment items that are well-suited for home use. Browse their catalog or web site and compare prices.

SAMPLE

To measure your progress, record your workouts. List the exercises you choose along with the resistance (or weight). Note the date and number of reps in the "day" columns. Change the exercises every 4-6 weeks.

	GROUP	EXERCISE	RESISTANCE	WEEK 1		WEEK 2		WEEK 3		WEEK 4	
				Day 1	Day 2	Day 1	Day 2	Day 1	Day 2	Day 1	Day 2
1	QUADS	Ball Squat	ball	18	18						
2	HAMSTRINGS	Leg Curl	5 lbs.	18	18						
3	SHINS	Toe Lift	none	14	18						
4	CALVES	Calf Raise	none	18	18						
5	CHEST	Chest Press	5 lbs.	15	17						
6	BACK	Pulldown	green tubing	18	18						
7	BICEPS	Arm Curl	5 lbs.	18	18						
8	TRICEPS	Pressdown	yellow tubing	15	18						
9	ABS	Crunch	ball	10	12						
10	LOW BACK	Opposite arm/leg lift	none	18	18						

	GROUP	EXERCISE	RESISTANCE	WEEK 1		WEEK 2		WEEK 3		WEEK 4	
				Day 1	Day 2	Day 1	Day 2	Day 1	Day 2	Day 1	Day 2
1	QUADS										
2	HAMSTRINGS										
3	SHINS										
4	CALVES										
5	CHEST										
6	BACK										
7	BICEPS										
8	TRICEPS										
9	ABS										
10	LOW BACK										

7
Stretch!
Quick and Easy Stretches for Busy People

> **The unbending tree is easily snapped.**
>
> *Lao Tzu,* Tao Te Ching

Welcome to the best, and often most neglected, part of any workout—stretching. Stretching is important because it helps to improve and maintain flexibility. It gives our bodies the ability to move freely, without stiffness. A good stretching routine can also help prevent or reduce injuries. Because it is often considered the relaxing component of a workout, stretching may help you to simply feel good and increase your enjoyment of cruising.

My favorite workout is one I call the "sunset stretch." It starts out with a two or three mile cruise, which I time so I finish about 20 minutes prior to sunset. This cruise takes place on the strand (walking path) along the coastline of Manhattan Beach in Southern California. During the cruise, I reflect on my day, think about things for which I am grateful and observe people enjoying life.

Just as I finish the cruise and daily meditation, I walk out onto the pier, heading straight into the sunset. This is my five-minute cruising cool-down which also serves as my stretching warm-up. Keep in mind, warm muscles help to make stretching more effective and may reduce your risk of injury. With about 15 minutes to go before sunset, I begin my stretching routine, focusing on all of the major muscle groups. With each stretch, I position my body so I am facing the sunset. The view gives me the chance to reflect, meditate and relax. It also guarantees that I will stretch at least 15 to 20 minutes. After all, there is no way I could walk away from the beauty of the sun touching down and sinking into the ocean.

Often, the length of my stretching session depends on how many times the color of the sky changes in the minutes following the sunset. For me, the sunset stretch is both a physical and spiritual experience.

Find the Perfect Place to Stretch

If you found a nice location to cruise, then finding an area where you can stretch and relax should be easy. Look for a place with natural beauty. Depending on where you live and what time of day you exercise, there are many options for finding the perfect setting for stretching. For many, a sunrise or sunset workout works well. Here are a few other suggestions:

- A nicely landscaped park
- On top of a hill, with city or country scenery
- Near a lake front, pond or park fountain

Besides nice scenery, look for a place that offers stretching aids, such as curbs, steps, park benches, fences, sign posts and railings. As you review the stretches presented in this chapter, you will learn how to use what is around you to help with your stretching.

Stretching Basics

Although there are various methods for stretching, the simplest and safest method for most people to understand and perform is called static stretching. Static stretching, also known as traditional stretching, occurs when you slowly stretch a muscle to the point of mild tension and then hold the stretch for 10 to 60 seconds. During the time you are holding the position, your body remains still. The key to this type of stretching is knowing how *mild* tension feels. Think of static stretching as the "stretch and hold" method.

> **Stretch after each cruising workout for a minimum of 10 minutes, preferably longer and more frequently if you have the time.**

Stretching after exercise helps to maintain and improve flexibility; however, be sure to cool down first from your cruising workout by walking slowly for a minimum of five minutes. As your cruises get longer, so must the cool-down time before you stretch. For example, after a half or full marathon, stretch *only* after cooling down by walking slowly for at least 30 minutes.

You may also incorporate some stretching into your cruising warm-up, just be sure to prepare your body for stretching by walking or jogging lightly for three to five minutes. Remember, muscles and joints that are warm are better-prepared for activity.

> **Stretch to the point of MILD tension.**

Once you have held the stretch for a while (10-60 seconds), the tension in the muscle should disappear. Every stretch should be comfortable. Do not force a stretch or take it to the point of severe discomfort where you really "feel it." This will cause your body to tighten up, thus fighting the stretch and risking injury. Only a relaxed muscle can be safely and comfortably stretched.

Hold each stretch for 10 to 60 seconds.

Be sure to avoid "bouncing" which can lead to injury. If you are not very flexible or haven't done much stretching on a regular basis, start with a 10-second hold and progress gradually to 30 seconds or longer as you become more familiar with the stretches. For muscles used during cruising workouts or areas where you feel tight, hold the stretches slightly longer or repeat the stretch two to three times. It is especially important for cruisers to thoroughly stretch the legs, hips and back.

Stretch carefully and correctly.

Look at each of the stretches in this chapter and focus on using the correct form. Always check your posture and body alignment. If you are unfamiliar with stretching, try the stretches first in front of a mirror to check your technique.

Breathe normally.

Breathing is important when stretching as it helps your body to relax. Some experts recommend you exhale as you ease into a stretch, which may help to release tension in your muscles; however, many people get confused when it comes to breathing techniques. The easiest guideline to remember is simply to breathe normally and avoid holding your breath.

The Pier Stretches

Whether performing these stretches on a pier looking into a sunset or anywhere else, the following stretches are a basic part of the cruising program. Most of these stretches, which for convenience, are performed in the standing position, focus on stretching the major muscle groups. If you hold each of these stretches for about 30 seconds, it should take you only ten minutes to complete the stretching workout.

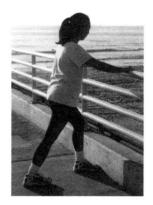

CALF STRETCH

7-1 Keep feet parallel and hip-width apart. Bend front knee and lean hips forward slightly to feel the stretch in the back of your lower leg.

HAMSTRING & CALF

HAMSTRING STRETCH

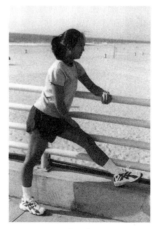

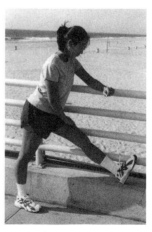

7-3 Slowly flex foot, pulling toes toward shin to feel stretch in rear thigh and rear lower leg muscles.

7-2 Keep back straight and lean forward slightly to feel stretch in rear thigh muscles.

THIGH STRETCH

7-4 Stand up straight with a neutral spine. Keep knees side by side. Press hip bones forward to feel stretch in the front thigh.

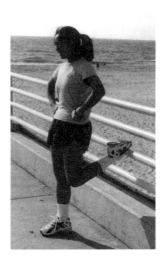

BACK STRETCHES

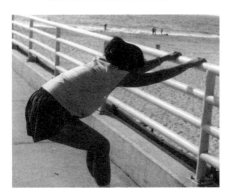

7-5A Be sure to have a firm grip on railing or other object. Keep back straight. Stretches spine, shoulders and arms.

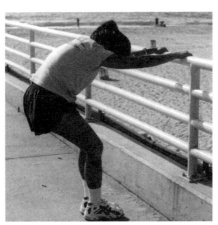

7-5B Round back and tuck chin to chest to feel stretch in upper back as well as spine and shoulders.

HIP STRETCH

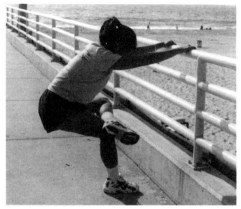

7-6 Cross one leg over thigh. Keep back straight and bend knee slightly to feel stretch in outer hip muscles. Be sure to have a firm grip on railing or other sturdy object.

CHEST STRETCH

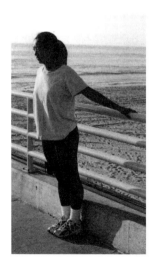

7-7 Keep back straight, head up and relax shoulders. Lean forward gently to feel stretch in the chest, shoulders and arms.

Safety Tip

When gripping railings, fences or other objects, be sure they are secure and dry. Be sure to have a firm grip at all times.

The Park Stretches

If you have some additional time, get down on the grass or your living room floor and include these key stretches to stretch your back, hips and legs.

HAMSTRING STRETCH
(with post)

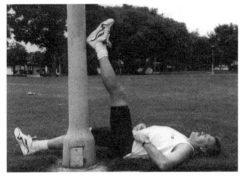

7-8 Use a pole, fence post or doorway. Keep a neutral spine with hips touching the ground. Relax foot and keep knee straight. Stretches the rear thigh muscles.

KNEES TO CHEST STRETCH

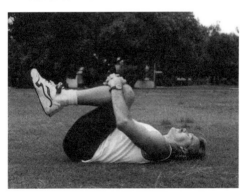

7-9 Relax upper body. Bring knees close to chest to feel stretch in back and buttocks.

SINGLE KNEE TO CHEST

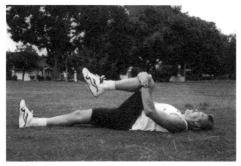

7-10 Keep lower back touching ground. Bring opposite knee close to chest to stretch the back and front hip muscles.

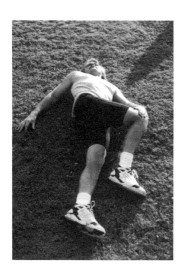

KNEE CROSSOVER

7-11 Keep shoulders on ground. Gently guide knee across body and over other leg to feel stretch in the outer hip, back, waist and chest (when arm is extended out to side). Note: knee does not have to touch ground.

Stretching Tip

When doing stretches that involve rotation of the spine (twisting), be sure to stretch only as far as comfortable for your body, avoiding excessive or forced twisting. Remember, only relaxed muscles can be safely stretched.

KNEELING BACK STRETCH

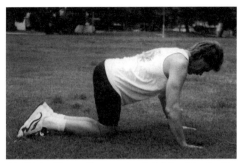

7-12A Keep elbows straight (not locked) and back, head and neck in a neutral position.

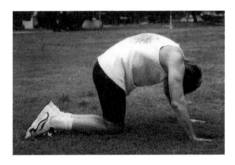

7-12B Round back and tuck chin to chest to stretch the back.

Active Stretches for Cruisers

Active stretching occurs when you tighten the opposing muscle group of the one you want to stretch without applying any resistance. For example, if you want to stretch your hamstring muscles behind your upper thigh, then you will need to contract (tighten) your quadriceps muscles in the front of your thigh, which causes the hamstrings to relax. Remember, only a relaxed muscle can be safely and effectively stretched. When performing active stretches, it is not necessary to hold the stretch for a certain period of time. Instead, you wait until you feel the muscle tension release. There is a learning process involved with active stretching. Try a few of these and see if you can determine when that muscle release occurs.

ACTIVE HAMSTRING & CALF

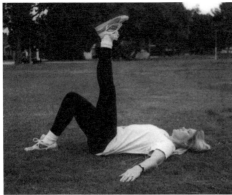

7-13A Keep leg being stretched, straight. Relax foot. Maintain a neutral spine. Back of thigh is stretched while front thigh is strengthened.

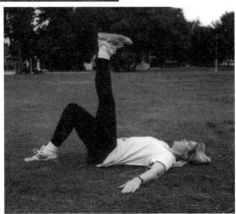

7-13B Pull toes toward shin to stretch the calf muscles.

ILIOTIBIAL BAND STRETCH

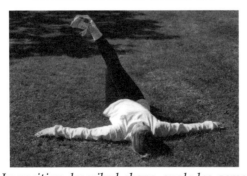

7-14 In position described above, angle leg across body while keeping entire back and hips on the ground. Point toes toward ground to feel stretch along the outside of the leg.

ACTIVE HAMSTRING & CALF
(with bent-knee start)

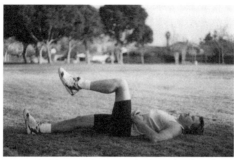

7-15A Keep thigh vertical and relax foot.

7-15B Slowly extend leg until mild stretch is felt in back of upper thigh. Keep a neutral spine position.

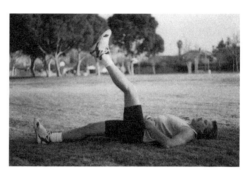

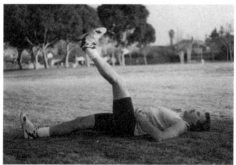

7-15C Pull toes toward shin to stretch calf. Keep thigh vertical. Note: Those who are less flexible do not need to extend the leg fully to feel these stretches.

Hold active stretches until tension in the stretched muscle disappears.

ACTIVE SEATED CALF

7-16 Keep back and legs straight. Slowly pull toes toward shins to feel stretch in calves.

Keep Stretching

If you truly want to feel good and improve your flexibility, stretch at least two days a week for 30 to 60 minutes in addition to your ten minutes of cool-down stretching. Check out the following resources if you want to learn more about stretching and flexibility training.

The Complete Idiot's Guide to Healthy Stretching by Chris Verna and Steve Hosid—Alpha Books, New York, NY

Comments: This book shows you how to find time for stretching in your daily routine and presents programs for various sports. It is an informative, basic guide to stretching which is fun to read, practical and easy to understand.

The Wharton's Stretch Book by Jim and Phil Wharton Times Books/Random House, New York, NY

Comments: This book focuses on active-isolated stretching and presents stretches for different sports and every-day activities. Sections on stretching during pregnancy and stretching for specific occupational activities are also included.

8
Nutrition and Weight Loss
Getting Back to the Simple Basics

> What really matters is what you do most of the time, not what you do occasionally. I call this the 80/20 approach: Do what you know you're supposed to 80% of the time; the other 20% of the time do whatever you want to!
>
> *Daniel Kosich, Ph.D.*
> *Get Real: A Personal Guide to Weight Management*

Stacie, one of my youngest clients at 15 years old, was full of questions about nutrition and weight loss. Fortunately, since we were cruising partners, I had plenty of time to teach her the basics of good nutrition. My challenge was to keep it simple enough so she could continue to enjoy eating while I desperately tried to shelter her from the poisonous nutrition and weight loss myths that seemed to be circling the halls of her high school.

I started by teaching Stacie the basics. Each week we focused on learning a different food group and how to improve our choices within that group. After six weeks, she had a basic understanding of the food groups and began applying what she had learned. After about six months, Stacie lost 15 pounds. I thought about all the other clients I have trained and suddenly realized that, although my program does not focus on weight loss, most of my clients have shed 10 to 20 pounds as a result of focusing on better eating habits and good nutrition. Could the secret be simplicity?

Have you ever heard the expression "you are what you eat?" Well, it's true. How you choose to fuel your body (with food) ultimately affects your health and well-being. When you are sick, does your doctor recommend potato chips, soda, cookies and fast food? Of course not. Usually the advice is chicken soup, juices and wholesome foods. What does that tell you? Generally, when you eat well, you feel well. That is, when your body is properly nourished it can provide you with energy, strengthen your immune system and help you feel and look your best.

Good nutrition is important for promoting health and lowering the risk for certain diseases, but when it comes to healthy eating, it is easy to become confused. We are always hearing about new diets and pills that promise weight loss. We read articles about good and bad foods. We watch news highlights of nutrition and medical miracles. We are led to believe there is a magic answer. With so much media hype and misleading information, does anyone really know how to eat well and lose weight safely?

When I introduce my clients to cruising, I always emphasize the importance of eating well. Since nutrition and physical activity go hand in hand, healthy eating is an essential part of the cruising program. In order for your body to get stronger physically, it needs proper nourishment.

The information presented in this chapter is intended to provide you with the basics of good nutrition. Once you have this foundation of knowledge, you will know how to gradually improve your eating habits and safely lose weight (if necessary). You will also learn some valuable sports nutrition tips to keep your body feeling its best during workouts.

Eating Essentials

Eating well is not as hard as you may think. There are three "essentials" to keep in mind when making food choices. Nancy Clark, R.D. cites these as the three basic keys to healthful eating in her *Sports Nutrition Guidebook*.

Variety

Eat different foods every day to get all the nutrients and other substances needed for good health. The more foods you like, the more nutritious and enjoyable your diet. If you are eating the same foods day after day, even healthful items, you may be missing out on some important nutrients. For example, you may have made the switch from a doughnut and coffee to a bagel and an orange for breakfast which is a step in the right direction. But if you have a bagel and orange every day for breakfast and have made similar changes at other meals, you may miss out on some important nutrients. Although eating the same foods day after day simplifies shopping and decision-making, it is not optimal for feeling nourished and energized. Variety across all food groups is necessary for optimal nutrition.

Moderation

Moderation means avoiding extremes. It is unrealistic to assume that one can eat perfectly healthy all the time. Rather than eliminating foods you enjoy, practice moderation. Even cookies, chips and soda can fit into a healthful diet. These foods are part of enjoying life and should not be considered "bad." Holidays and celebrations featuring high fat foods and lots of sweets are also a part of life in many cultures. Use common sense and portion control and any food you love can be part of a healthy diet.

Use the 80/20 rule as a guide for moderation. This means making healthy choices about 80 percent of the time and working in "fun" and perhaps "not so healthy" food choices the other 20 percent of time. When it comes to health, it's not what you do for short periods that really makes the difference. It is what you do most of the time (80 percent) over the course of your life that matters. The 80/20 rule also works well with other aspects of your health such as exercise and attitude.

Wholesomeness Whenever possible, choose foods that are minimally processed and have few or no additives. For example, choose whole wheat rather than white bread; fresh fruits rather than fruit juices; fresh vegetables rather than fried vegetables (onion rings, potato chips). Diluted, unsweetened fruit juices, low or nonfat milk and water are better beverage choices than soda or high-sugar juice drinks. As a general rule, avoid foods that have a long list of ingredients you are unfamiliar with or cannot pronounce. Wholesome foods generally have more nutrients, so choose them as often as possible.

Know the Basics

Before you can begin to understand nutrition or weight loss, you must first have a simple understanding of basic nutrition. Once you know this, you can apply this knowledge and common sense to evaluate diets, eating plans or hyped headlines.

There are six basic nutrients necessary for health: carbohydrates, fats, proteins, vitamins, minerals and water. The foods we eat are made up of various combinations of these nutrients, in different proportions. For example, an orange, which is mostly carbohydrate, contains just over one gram of protein and about a half a gram of fat along with its vitamins, minerals and water.

When a food item is classified as being primarily a carbohydrate, fat or protein, keep in mind that usually refers to the food's highest percentage of a nutrient. Good health requires all of these nutrients in proper balance. First, let's take a look at each nutrient and its function in the body. Later in the chapter I'll provide you with simple guidelines to help you get the correct amounts in your diet.

Carbohydrates

Carbohydrates, also known as "carbs," are the main source of energy for all body functions including physical activity. Carbohydrates provide immediate energy and also help your body digest and absorb protein and fat. To avoid misinformation, when referring to carbohydrates, it is important to understand the difference between simple and complex carbohydrates.

Simple carbohydrates generally enter your bloodstream quickly and provide immediate energy. These types of carbohydrates, such as refined sugars and starches (cake, cookies, soda, sweetened fruit juices), usually contain a high number of calories and few nutrients. Complex carbohydrates are more like a time-release pill; they enter your bloodstream more slowly and provide you with more ongoing energy. Unlike simple carbohydrates, complex carbohydrates, such as fruits, vegetables and grains, also provide vitamins and minerals and should make up the foundation of a healthful diet.

Fats

Fats provide us with the most concentrated source of energy in the diet; twice the amount of carbohydrates. Fats also help with the absorption of certain vitamins, A, D, E and K. Like carbohydrates, there are two types of fats: saturated and unsaturated. Saturated fats, which, except for coconut oils, are found mainly in animal products, become hard at room temperature, while unsaturated fats remain liquid. For good health, it is important to limit the total amount of fat in your diet, especially saturated fat which has been linked to heart disease and certain cancers.

Excess fat can also cause weight gain. For this reason, many people have gone to extremes to cut all fat from their diets. This is not wise since our bodies need some fat. Ironically, Vitamin E, which is found in some high-fat foods such as vegetable oils, nuts and seeds, helps protect us from heart disease. Fat also helps keep our hair and skin looking great. So yes, we do need some fat, but try to keep the "moderation" concept in mind.

Proteins

Protein is the major source of building material for all body tissues including muscles, blood, skin and vital organs such as the heart and brain. It is an important element for a healthy immune system and is also needed to make up many of the body's hormones, which control a variety of body functions. When there are insufficient amounts of carbohydrates and fats in the diet, protein may also be used as a source of energy.

Protein provides the body with amino acids, which help to build body tissues, and many amino acids are made by your body. Those that are not are called "essential" amino acids because you need to get them through your diet. When a food provides all the essential amino acids, it is called a "complete protein." Animal foods provide complete proteins, however, some legumes (beans and peas) and grains will provide all the essential amino acids when combined.

The recreational exerciser needs about a half gram of protein per pound of body weight. Any excess dietary protein will be stored as fat since the body does not consider protein a main source for energy. You need mostly carbohydrates in your diet, then fats, then protein. Making a high-protein food a side dish rather than the main course will ensure you don't get too much.

Vitamins & Minerals

Vitamins and minerals are needed by our bodies in small amounts and help with a variety of body functions. Vitamins, which are organic substances found in all plants and animals, help build body tissues, prevent nutritional deficiency diseases and make it possible for your body to produce energy from food. Minerals are inorganic substances found in non-living things such as rocks and soil, but are also found in plants (which get minerals from soil) and animals (who eat plants). Minerals combine to form structures of the body such as bones (calcium) and red blood cells (iron). Although vitamins and minerals work together in proper balance and help your body produce energy, they are not a direct source of energy.

If you eat a varied diet consisting of healthful and wholesome foods, you should get all the vitamins and minerals you need. But when you consider our polluted environment, busy lives, attraction to fast and convenience foods, varied tastes and stressful world, it is easy to see how nutritional deficiencies can occur. Even exercise, when taken to extremes, can break the body down, making it necessary to consider taking vitamin and mineral supplements. Although it is best to get your nutrients through food, a standard, one-a-day multivitamin/mineral supplement may provide some additional protection against deficiencies.

Water

Water is essential for life. A person can live for weeks without food, but only a few days without water. Our bodies are about 60 to 75 percent water, making it the main element of the fluids that are within and around all living cells. Water helps regulate body temperature and fluid balance, transport nutrients, including oxygen, and is a part of all body functions. Proper hydration is especially important for moderate exercisers who can lose water through sweating.

During exercise, especially sessions lasting over one hour, a lack of water can cause muscle cramps, nausea and dehydration. It is important to drink enough water before, during and after exercise.

Plan With The Pyramid

Now you know the six basic nutrients. When it comes to how much of each, it is easy to become confused. The general recommendation for a sensible diet is 60-65% carbohydrates, 20-25% fat and about 10-15% protein. Without tracking the carbohydrates, fats and protein in everything you eat and then doing some math, how is the average person supposed to know when they have eaten a balanced diet?

The Food Guide Pyramid was developed by the US Department of Agriculture to help make it easier for people to eat a balanced diet. If you follow the guidelines for how many servings to eat in each of the six food groups, it's likely that you'll be within the recommended percentages. The only thing you need to do is become familiar with serving sizes of foods.

Unlike calorie-counting and food-logging, serving size education is an easy and practical way to begin to eat more sensibly. The Food Guide Pyramid is made up of five major food groups and a sixth group from which you should eat sparingly. Follow the guidelines for the recommended number of daily servings from each group and keep the 80/20 approach in mind when using the pyramid.

- Choose most of your foods from the grain products, vegetable and fruit groups.

- Eat moderate amounts of foods from the milk and meat and beans groups.

- Choose sparingly foods that provide few nutrients and are high in fat and sugars.

The Food Guide Pyramid

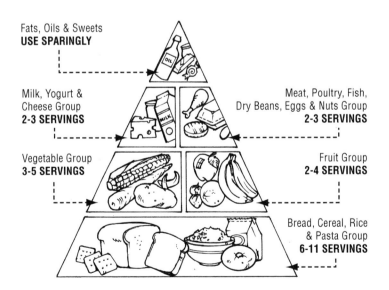

The pyramid makes it easier to monitor your daily calorie intake without counting calories. On the pyramid, a range is given for servings for each food group. Shoot for the lower number if you want to take in about 1600 calories a day (not many people should be below this level, especially those who exercise). The higher number in the range represents about 2800 daily calories. For better nutrition, pay attention to both the quality and quantity of the foods you select. You will get more vitamins, minerals and other beneficial substances by striving for higher-quality food items. Refer to food labels to help determine serving sizes and to evaluate the quality.

Understanding The Pyramid Week by Week

Changing all of your habits at once is nearly impossible. I suggest the week-by-week approach to my clients who want to learn how to eat better. Focus on evaluating your current eating habits and making better choices within each food group one week at a time. In six weeks, you will have made it through all of the food groups without becoming overwhelmed. This is an easy and practical approach to learning the Food Guide Pyramid.

Week 1
The Grainy Foundation

At the base of the pyramid is the **Grain Products Group (bread, cereal, rice and pasta) .** The recommendation is **6 - 11 servings** a day. For the first week, try measuring your servings, especially rice and pasta. It is an eye-opening experience that will help you realize how easy it is to overeat from this group and help you understand why high-carbohydrate foods have gotten a bad rap. For weight loss, keep to six servings a day and for peak performance or if you are a larger person (men), go for 11 servings daily.

Here are some examples of one serving:

1 slice of bread
1 small muffin or roll
½ hamburger or hot dog bun
4-6 small crackers
1 four-inch pancake
2 rice cakes
1 tortilla
3 cups popcorn
12 small pretzels
½ cup of cooked cereal, rice or pasta
1 cup dry cereal
½ bagel or English muffin

During the week, strive for higher quality in this food group:

- Choose whole grain breads, crackers and cereals rather than those made with refined white flour ("whole wheat" should be one of the first ingredients). Look for whole wheat English muffins—they make great mini pizzas!

- Some health food stores carry whole wheat breaded fish filets, frozen pot pies and sandwich pockets with wheat crust and wide variety of whole grain snacks.

- Try carrot, spinach or whole wheat pastas.

- If you do not like brown rice, try mixing it with white rice for a nutritious boost.

- Select cereals low in fat and sugar, such as oatmeal, shredded wheat and bran.

- This food group also includes cakes, cookies, doughnuts and pastries, but since these foods are high in fat and sugar, they fit better in the Fats, Oils and Sweets group.

Week 2
Strive For Five

Just above the grain products group, which makes up the base of the pyramid, sits the **Vegetable Group**. Strive for **3-5 servings** a day. If you are going to eat too much of anything, vegetables are the best choice. Most are low in fat and calories and high in fiber, vitamins and minerals. My nutrition professor once told me that a vegetable is technically defined as a root, stem or leaf of a plant. So eggplants, tomatoes and peppers are actually fruits! Try to eat more vegetables of the root (carrots, potatoes), stem (celery, broccoli) and leaf (lettuce, spinach, cabbage) variety. But go ahead and consider the other "vegetable-fruits" as vegetables to avoid confusion. Here is what counts as one serving:

1 cup of raw leafy vegetables
½ cup cooked or raw vegetables
¾ cup of vegetable juice
Lettuce and tomato (on a sandwich)
½ cup tomato sauce
1 medium carrot

Keeping track of your vegetable intake this week will help you realize that most people do not eat enough vegetables. Here are some tips for adding more vegetables to your diet:

• Buy some frozen vegetarian entrees such as vegetable lasagna, veggie pot pies or baked potatoes with vegetables.

• Have a green salad every day. Use dark leafy greens such as spinach and dark green lettuce. Be careful about the salad dressing. If you prefer regular salad dressing to low or nonfat dressings, limit your serving to one tablespoon and toss the salad well.

- Have carrot and celery sticks at least twice during the week with a sandwich.

- Juices count! If you don't like mixed vegetable juice, try a shot or two of carrot or wheat grass juice.

- Make one meal a day vegetarian. Try grilled or stir-fried vegetables over a half cup of rice or pasta. Frozen vegetable side dishes that you can pop in the microwave make great lunches and are usually low in fat and calories (even when you eat the whole package).

Week 3
Two For Two

Right beside the vegetable group and equally important is the **Fruit Group.** Fruits and vegetables provide us with a quality source of carbohydrates, vitamins and minerals. The recommendation is **2 - 4 servings** a day. Fruits make an excellent snack, so this week while you are focusing on fruits, try replacing two of your regular snacks with two fruit snacks. Whole, fresh fruits are usually low in fat and high in nutrients and also make a great dessert. Here are some examples of one serving:

1 medium apple, banana, peach, plum, pear or orange
½ cup of cooked or canned fruit
¾ cup of fruit juice
1 cup of raspberries, blueberries, strawberries, grapes or cherries
½ grapefruit
2 tablespoons raisins

This week, place a bowl with five different pieces of washed whole fruit on your desk at work or in your refrigerator. Set a goal of eating one piece a day which takes care of half your fruit requirement. If Friday comes along and you still have 4 pieces left, then eat them all for lunch. Here are some other suggestions for eating more fruits:

- Try bananas, apples, oranges, pears and raisins for quick and easy snacks.

- Prepare fruits, such as melons, grapes, pineapple and berries by washing them and placing them in ready-to-eat storage containers.

- Fruit juices count as fruit servings; however, some juices are high in sugar. If you choose to drink fruit juices, try diluting them with water to decrease calorie and sugar content.

- Select fresh fruit topped with light whipped cream for desserts.

Week 4
Got Milk?

The **Milk Group (milk, yogurt and cheese)** sits above the vegetable group and since it's closer to the top of the pyramid, it has a smaller number of recommended daily servings. You should eat moderate amounts from the milk group, **2-3 servings a day,** to be sure you are getting key nutrients such as calcium, phosphorus and protein.

Milk and milk products are important part of good nutrition; however, some individuals are "lactose intolerant." This means that their bodies have trouble digesting lactose, a sugar found in milk products. Yogurt may be a better choice for these individuals since the lactose is already broken down, relieving the body of that function.

In the milk group, here is what counts as one serving:

1 cup of milk or yogurt (8 ounces)
1½ ounces of natural cheese
2 ounces of processed cheese
3 tablespoons grated cheese
½ cup of cottage cheese
¼ cup of shredded cheese
the cheese on 1 medium slice of pizza
1 cup of ice cream

This week, try switching to lower fat products from this group and cutting back on cheese.

- If you drink whole milk (which is 4% fat by volume), try 2% or mix your whole milk with low or nonfat milk.

- Try different low-fat yogurts, but be careful of those with a lot of added sugar (such as frozen yogurt)

- Cut back on cheese; it's loaded with fat. While very small amounts provide important nutrients, it's easy to go overboard with cheese. Fat-free varieties are often taste-free as well, so try reduced-fat cheese instead. If you like pizza, order it with less cheese and more veggies, then limit your portion to one or two slices.

If you do not consume foods from the milk group, you'll need to get your calcium from other foods such as tofu, dark leafy greens, broccoli, beans, salmon or orange juice fortified with calcium. While ice cream is a good source of calcium, keep in mind it is high in fat, sugar and calories. If you love ice cream, eat it only occasionally and keep your portions small.

Week 5
Protein Power

Right next to the Milk Group on the pyramid sits the **Meat and Beans Group (meat, poultry, fish, dry beans, eggs and nuts).** The recommendation is **2-3 servings** a day. While foods from the milk group provide some protein, foods from the Meat and Beans Group provide the highest percentage. But be careful, it's easy to go overboard because many foods in this group are high in fat and calories. Here is what counts as one serving:

2-3 ounces of cooked lean meat, poultry or fish
    (about the size of a deck of cards)
1 pork or veal chop,¾ inch thick
½ chicken breast
2 thin slices of roasted meat
1 medium meat patty (beef, turkey or chicken)
¾ cup of tuna, salmon or crab
15 large shrimp or 18 oysters

The following counts as ***one ounce*** *of meat:*
½ cup cooked beans or 1 egg
2 tablespoons of peanut butter
¼ cup nuts or seeds

Some people prefer to calculate their protein needs in grams rather than servings. A general recommendation for the adult recreational exerciser is a half gram of protein per pound of body weight. During the week, count the grams of protein you eat daily. You can use food labels or purchase a small book listing grams of protein in common foods. Are you getting enough or too much protein? Chances are you are getting too much and remember, protein is not generally used as an energy source, so any excess may be converted to fat!

Week 6
Spare Me!

At the top of the pyramid is the **Fats, Oils and Sweets Group**. There are no recommendations for servings in this group other than to consume foods from this group **sparingly.** Many of the high-fat or high-sugar foods from some of the other groups really belong here. If you eat foods from this group, you should do so in moderation. Here is what might be considered a serving:

1 or 2 small cookies
1 thin slice of cake or ½ doughnut
3-5 pieces of hard candy or ½ candy bar
2-3 small pieces of chocolate
2 teaspoons of sugar
2 tablespoons syrup
½ cup ice cream
½ can of soda
1-2 tablespoons of oil (for a stir-fry)

You don't need to eliminate these foods entirely. If you do, you may find yourself wanting them more. Birthdays, parties and holidays are a fun part of life. Enjoy high-fat and high-sugar foods only occasionally and in very small portions. This week, keep track of all your fats, sweets and oils (or high fat foods). At the end of the week ask yourself if you ate these foods in moderation. Your common sense will steer you toward the correct answer.

If you eat these foods in excess, start by cutting back gradually. For example, if you have a regular soda every day, try drinking a half a can of soda instead. Or if you have a candy bar every day, switch to one every other day. Small but consistent changes in your habits have a large impact on how your body feels and looks.

A Few More Quick Tips for Good Nutrition

Establish consistent eating habits, including breakfast every morning. If you don't have time for a breakfast meal, grab a banana, yogurt, a glass of orange juice or munch on a handful of dry cereal to get you going. This is especially important if you exercise in the morning. You need some food to give you an energy boost and prevent feeling light-headed during your workout. Eat regularly throughout the day and do not skip meals. If you are not hungry, eat a smaller meal or healthy snack instead.

If you drink alcoholic beverages, do so in moderation. One drink per day for women and two for men is considered moderate. Here is what counts as one drink:

> *12 ounces of regular beer (150 calories)*
> *5 ounces of wine (100 calories)*
> *1 ounce of 80-proof distilled spirits (100 calories)*

Some people should not drink alcoholic beverages at all. These include:

- Children and adolescents

- Individuals who cannot keep their drinking moderate or who have a family history of alcohol-related problems

- Pregnant women or those trying to conceive

- Anyone who plans to drive or do other activities that require attention or skill (including sports and exercise)

- Those taking medications, prescription or other

- Individuals with any serious health issues

- Those trying to lose weight

Drink plenty of water. Try for 6-8 glasses each day (about 2 quarts). Drink more in hot weather and when exercising. If you can't tolerate the taste of plain water, try diluting juice drinks (half and half). This way you'll save some calories and increase your water intake at the same time.

Eating Well: The Easiest Way to Weight Loss

If you follow the week by week guidelines for learning how to eat better using the food guide pyramid, you may already be on your way to weight loss (a side-effect of better eating). Nutritious eating combined with a few helpful tips for weight loss can help you achieve or maintain your healthy weight. The information presented in this chapter is designed to help you understand how to lose weight and apply some simple guidelines for making it happen.

The best way to lose weight (i.e., body fat) is through a combination of exercise and sensible, nutritious eating. Diets don't work. What does work is making small changes in your eating and exercise habits. Over time, this gives you the best, long-lasting results.

In spite of all the "new" diets and weight loss programs that we hear about, there is really one simple, no-fail way to lose weight: **exercise a little more and eat a little less**. This method works nearly 100% of the time. The goal of weight loss is to use up more total calories than you take in.

A pound of fat is equal to about 3500 calories. When you have burned up an extra 3500 calories, usually over the course of a week or two, a pound of fat is lost. This can be done by eating about 250 calories less each day and burning up about 250 calories more each day. To understand this, let's take a look at the energy equation.

The Energy Equation

Eating provides your body with energy through calories (a calorie is a unit of energy). You need this energy to sustain life since everything you do, even sleeping, requires energy (i.e., burns calories).

Calories in $<$ Calories out $=$ Fat loss
Calories in $>$ Calories out $=$ Fat gain
Calories in $=$ Calories out $=$ Maintenance

The energy equation can help you understand why it is impossible for your body to lose 10 pounds of fat in one week. If you did lose 10 pounds of weight in one week, you can bet that most of what you lost was water and lean tissue (muscle and bone). This type of weight loss sets you up for fast weight gain, usually in the form of more fat.

Realistically, it is not practical to count calories and most people don't want to bother. Focus on eating well first, according to the food guide pyramid. Most of my clients have lost weight simply by eating better and focusing on the following helpful weight loss tips:

Eat smaller portions. This is the easiest way to lose weight without drastically changing your lifestyle. You may need to measure foods and read labels for about a week or so to become more aware of portion sizes. For many this is the key to weight loss. Most of my clients just ate less and since they were cruising, they were exercising more. It worked!

Cut back (don't eliminate). If you love chips, cookies or chocolate, try cutting back your portion each time you have this food item. By cutting *back* instead of cutting *out*, you are less likely to feel deprived. For example, one of my clients who had been trying to lose weight for years, simply reduced wine to only special occasions and lost 18 pounds! She found that when she had a glass of wine, she was more likely to "munch" and overeat. Cutting back was the answer for her.

Eat foods lower in fat. Fat has twice the calories of carbohydrates and protein. Although your body needs fat in small amounts, try to make one or more low fat food choice each day—substitute a piece of fruit for a bag of chips.

Keep a 7 day journal of everything you eat. This can help you become more aware of what you are eating and where you can cut back. Look at your food journal at the end of the week and ask yourself, did I follow the guidelines? Is there any place I can cut back?

Try to understand the difference between physical hunger and emotional hunger. Although this topic is beyond the scope of this book, if you eat for emotional reasons (boredom, anxiety, stress, etc.), try to find a way to keep yourself busy. One of my clients paints her nails when she is watching television and says it helps prevent her from eating out of boredom. Ask yourself if there is there anything you can do when you are bored that might prevent you from eating.

Be patient! Making small changes in lifetime habits *is* the magic everyone has been looking for. You may not always be able to follow the guidelines for good nutrition and/or weight loss, but you'll find if you strive for progress, not perfection, you will be on the road to better health.

Fueling Your Workouts

Proper nutrition before, during and after your cruising workouts is important. What you eat can affect your performance. Here are some general tips for eating before, during and after exercise.

- For workouts over one hour, eat at least an hour before to allow adequate time for digestion. Choose high-carbohydrate foods such as oranges, grapefruits, apples, pears, bananas, milk, yogurt, spaghetti, rice, oatmeal, beans (legumes) and corn. These foods help provide sustained energy.

- Allow enough time for your meals to digest. Generally, allow 3-4 hours for a large meal, 2-3 for a small meal and 1-2 hours for a liquid meal or small snack. Everyone is different so you may have to experiment with pre-exercise meal planning.

- If you think you may become too anxious to eat before an event (whether it is a 10K race or a marathon), be sure to eat well the day before. Eat a healthy dinner and an extra snack before bed.

- Do not try new or unfamiliar foods before an event. Instead, try them during training sessions so you will learn what works best for you.

- During the event, especially lengthy endurance events such as a half or full marathon, some people need and can tolerate small amounts of food. High-carbohydrate foods that quickly enter into your bloodstream can help give you some immediate energy. A few examples are sport drinks, fruit juices, jelly beans, bagels, crackers, glucose gels or tablets.

- Always drink plenty of water before during and after exercise to prevent dehydration. Beginning 24 hours before endurance exercise, drink 4-8 ounces of fluid each waking hour, 16 ounces up to two hours before and 4-8 ounces 5-10 minutes before. During exercise, drink 8-10 ounces every 15-20 minutes. If the weather is hot, drink as often as you can.

- When you are hydrating your body it is important to avoid fluids such as alcohol and caffeinated beverages which can work against what you are trying to accomplish. Water is generally considered best; however, some research shows that diluting sport drinks or orange juice may help certain minerals such as potassium and sodium to be absorbed better by the body.

- When rehydrating your body after a long event, it can sometimes take up to 24 hours to replenish fluids. Continue to take in fluids and avoid alcohol (which is dehydrating).

- After a half or full marathon, be sure to keep yourself in the recovery mode. Continue to replenish fluids and make healthy food choices. This recovery period is critical for helping to increase immune function and may be the most important part of the process. Sure you can have that slice of pizza, but don't resort to replenishing your body with junk. Instead power up with fresh fruit or vegetable juices, pasta, soup and dark green leafy salads. It is not uncommon for people to catch colds or other viruses after an endurance event.

Keep in mind, everyone is different. What works for one may not for someone else. To find what food and fluid intake patterns work best for you, experiment during training sessions. And every time you have a great cruise, filled with energy, write down what you ate and drank before, during and after.

Summing it Up

I believe physical activity and good nutrition hold the key to health and longevity. Although nutrition can be confusing at times, try to keep the basics and common sense in mind. Lastly, be patient and you will be successful.

Resource Recommendations

The Sports Nutrition Guidebook by Nancy Clark
Human Kinetics, Champaign, IL

Comments: This book is for anyone who wants up-to-date food advice that is easy to understand and apply. It is one of the best resources for those who want to know how to eat to fuel an active lifestyle. Use as a reference or read it cover to cover. Either way, it's a great resource.

Nutrition For Dummies by Carol Ann Rinzler
IDG Books Worldwide, Foster City, CA

Comments: This book provides simple and practical nutrition advice. It gives the basics as well as everything you need to know about fad diets, food labels, eating out, food as medicine, appetite and much more. I especially like the easy-to-read format and the section on nutrition myths. This is a good, basic reference that will expand your nutrition knowledge.

Get Real: A Personal Guide to Weight Management by Daniel Kosich—Published by IDEA, San Diego, CA **www.ideafit.com**

> **Comments:** At last, a weight management approach you could live with. By far, this is one of the best weight loss books I've seen. I use it for the foundation of a weight management course I teach. It offers common sense, practical advice in three key areas: physical activity, sensible eating and self-empowerment. There is a wealth of good information packed into this easy-to-read weight loss guide. Many of my clients read it over and over, anytime they want to be brought back to the real world. It is well worth the investment!

Dietary Guidelines for Americans , Fourth Edition 1995, by the U.S. Department of Agriculture and the U.S. Department of Health and Human Services Ask for Home and Garden Bulletin No. 232 (It's free!) (202) 720-7327

> **Comments:** This is a free 40-page pamphlet which offers sound advice for healthy eating. It's brief and gives you seven dietary guidelines for good health. Nothing fancy, but all Americans should know and try to apply these basic guidelines.

Center For Science in the Public Interest (CSPI) is an independent, nonprofit consumer health group. CSPI supports honest food labeling and advertising, healthier foods in restaurants, pro-health alcohol policies, safer food additives and sustainable agriculture. CSPI, 1875 Connecticut Avenue N.W., Suite 300, Washington, DC 20009-5728 — **www.cspinet.org**

> **Comments:** CSPI publishes the Nutrition Action Healthletter which is a great way to keep yourself up-do-date with the hottest topics in nutrition. They also post a variety of information on their web site.

Cruising Q & A

Answers to Commonly Asked Questions

> Knowledge is power, but
> enthusiasm pulls the switch.
>
> *Ivern Ball*

1. I am starting with the Base Training program and I am definitely a non-exerciser. How long will it take before each workout gets easier?

Generally, any distance you complete becomes easier after three to four workouts. That is, if you are starting with a 2:3 cruise plan, the first time you do it, it will be somewhat challenging. After you repeat that cruise plan three to four times, it should feel easier. As a general rule, whenever a cruising workout feels difficult, switch to an easier cruise plan and stick with it until it feels comfortable. Apply this rule when you go on vacation, are ill or if you skip workouts. Also, keep in mind, that no matter how fit a person is, there will always be days that are just harder than others. That is a fact of exercise.

2. What if I want to exercise more than three days a week?

If you are not used to regular exercise, stay with three days a week until you have developed consistency. Three days is moderate and a realistic time commitment, especially for people with busy lives. You will be more likely to stick with your goals and enjoy exercise if you don't try to do too much. If you can remain consistent with the three workouts for at least four weeks, you may incorporate other activities on your "non-cruising" days.

Walking, cycling and swimming are excellent choices for additional heart and lung conditioning. Climbing stairs and hiking, while good exercises, use the same muscle groups as cruising; therefore, may be overworked which can lead to injury. You should consider adding some strength training to your exercise plan. A quick and effective strength routine is presented in Chapter 6. Stretching and Yoga are also excellent choices. To exercise consistently, the most important thing to remember is varying your choices and making them fit your lifestyle.

3. Should I exercise if the weather is bad?

Remember, cruising is designed to help you enjoy the outdoors. Use common sense when evaluating weather conditions. It can be fun splashing around in a little rain; challenging on a windy day and simply beautiful during a light snow. Try not to let bad weather stop you unless the conditions are severe or unhealthy (such as poor air quality), in which case you should postpone your workout or train indoors. Training through a variety of weather conditions will better prepare you for similar conditions should they occur during a race.

4. Should I exercise when I am sick?

Whether or not you should exercise when you are sick actually depends on how sick you are. It is *always* best to first check with your doctor. However, as a general rule for common colds and flu, if your symptoms are above the neck (such as a mild head cold), you can continue with exercise, but keep the workout easy. If your symptoms are from the neck down (persistent cough or body aches), take some time off and rest. Your body can't heal if all your energy is going to your workouts. Don't worry about losing any conditioning. Again, when in doubt, check with your doctor.

5. What if I don't know the distance where I am cruising?

For most of my clients, the distance programs have been shown to provide the best motivation. Telling your friends you completed six miles sounds more impressive than saying "I just cruised for an hour." However, there may be times when distance training may not be possible, such as when you are on vacation or in an unfamiliar area. Check out the time-based programs in the Appendix if you prefer to do all your training based on time. You will get the same results.

6. I've heard that you should train beyond the distance of the race you plan to run. Why don't you recommend that in your cruising programs?

All of my programs are intended for the first-timer whose goal is to finish. When you cruise a certain distance for the first time at an event, it is more exciting when the distance completed is a new personal record. Most, if not all, of my clients have felt their best upon crossing the finish line, knowing that the distance they just completed was a milestone that they were reaching for the very first time. It made receiving the finisher's medal even more exciting. For more experienced cruisers, training beyond the race distance may yield a better performance; however, in the case of a marathon, training beyond 26.2 miles takes its toll on the body. For some, a distance that long is too much to do more than once a year.

7. What does it mean when you get a pain in your side?

A sharp, sudden pain in your side just below your rib cage, also known as a "side stitch," can occur when you try to do too much too soon, when you are exercising at a high intensity or if you ate too close to your workout time. Side stitches are common among those who are just beginning an exercise program, but become more infrequent as you get in better shape. If you get a side stitch during a cruise, walk slowly. Take some deep breaths and massage the area with your fingers. The stitch will usually go away within a few minutes.

8. What if I get injured?

Little aches and pains are common from time to time, especially as your body adapts to the impact of running and walking. If you experience minor joint discomfort during your workout, modify your cruise plan to include more walking until the discomfort subsides. As a general rule, any ache or pain that goes away within a couple of days is usually nothing to worry about. Applying ice for 10-15 minutes will help reduce inflammation. Consult your physician if you experience any severe injury or pain. To prevent injuries, be sure to run on level surfaces and follow the cruising guidelines detailed in Chapter 2. A good book about injuries is recommended at the end of Chapter 5.

9. I'd like to bring my dog along on my cruises. Is there anything special I should consider?

Dogs need to be conditioned the same way as humans, slowly and gradually. But some breeds are better exercisers than others. First, check with your veterinarian for specific recommendations for the breed and age of your dog. The best time to bring your dog along is when you are starting the Base Training program or doing the marathon recovery program. Remember, dogs wear fur coats and can easily become overheated. Their feet can also be hurt by hot, concrete surfaces. Whenever training with your dog, stay with a cruise and keep the distance to no more than 2-3 miles at a time. Always clean up after your dog.

10. I am unable to do even small amounts of running but would like to try walking a 10K or a half-marathon. How would I modify the training program?

Any one of the cruising programs in this book can be followed by those who wish to do walking only. Simply complete the distance goals by walking instead of cruising. The same general guideline may be applied for those who wish to run without any walking, although I feel even experienced runners should take walking breaks.

The training schedules presented in this book are designed for busy people who have most of their free time on the weekends. This program has worked not only for cruisers, but also for walkers who have specific events they are training for. Whatever you choose to be your main activity, walking, running or cruising, be consistent and you'll see amazing results.

Afterword

The first step is up to you. I hope you choose to take it. If you do and if you stick with it, you will succeed. Hopefully, this book will guide you along the way. The goal is for you to experience the benefits of a physically active lifestyle and help you see that getting and staying in shape is a lot easier than most people realize. Of course you don't have to complete a marathon or even a half-marathon to "succeed" in this program, but achieving such a daunting physical challenge will do more for your self-confidence than you've ever imagined.

If you are successful and achieve your goal, whether it be general fitness or completing a half or full marathon, please let me know of your experience (see address and e-mail on copyright page). You will be an inspiration to others who may want *you* to show them the way. Be a mentor and take someone through this program. Not only will this keep you exercising and help you stay motivated, but you will get a tremendous sense of satisfaction from helping someone improve his or her health through physical activity. As the news spreads, more of us will choose to be active and lead healthier lives. This is my ultimate goal for this book.

Through your experience I hope you will learn that taking small steps can help you achieve any goal in life and that you cannot fail unless you give up.

> **Your own resolution to success is more important than any other one thing.**
>
> *Abraham Lincoln*

Appendix

Cruising Programs

Use the following cruising programs for personal tracking and training notes. If you do not know the distance where you are training, select a time-based program.

The Base Training Program

Mileage-Based Training

	Day One run:walk (minutes)	**Day Two** run:walk (minutes)	**Weekend** run:walk (minutes)
Week 1 1 mile	2:3	2:3	2:3
Week 2 1.5 miles	3:3	4:3	5:3
Week 3 2 miles	6:3	7:3	8:3
Week 4 2.5 miles	10:3	12:3	14:3
Week 5 3 miles	15:2	15:2	15:2
Week 6 3 miles	20:2	25:2	Try to run 3 miles without walking!

Training Notes:

_____

_____

_____

_____

_____

_____

The Base Training Program

Time-Based Training

Time	Day One *run:walk* *(minutes)*	Day Two *run:walk* *(minutes)*	Weekend *run:walk* *(minutes)*
Week 1 *10 min.*	2:3	2:3	2:3
Week 2 *15 min.*	3:3	4:3	5:3
Week 3 *20 min.*	6:3	7:3	8:3
Week 4 *25 min.*	10:3	12:3	14:3
Week 5 *30 min.*	15:2	15:2	15:2
Week 6 *35 min.*	20:2	25:2	Try to run 30 minutes without walking!

Training Notes:

_____

_____

_____

_____

_____

_____

The Half-Marathon Program

Mileage-Based Training

	Day One (run or cruise)		Day Two (run or cruise)		Weekend (cruise 10:2)	
	MILES	TIME	MILES	TIME	MILES	TIME
Week 1	3		3		4	
Week 2	3		3		5	
Week 3	3		3		6	
Week 4 (easy)	3		3		7	
Week 5	3		3		8	
Week 6	3		3		9	
Week 7	3		3		10	
Week 8 (easy)	3		3		6 (hills)	
Week 9	3		3 (hills)		12	
Week 10 (easy)	3		3		6 (hills)	
Week 11	3		3 (hills)		6	
Week 12	3		3		13.1 Half-marathon	

Training Notes:

_____

_____

_____

_____

_____

The Half-Marathon Program

Time-Based Training

	Day One *(run or cruise)*	Day Two *(run or cruise)*	Weekend *(cruise 10:2)*
	TIME (minutes)	TIME (minutes)	TIME (minutes)
Week 1	30-35	30-35	45
Week 2	30-35	30-35	55
Week 3	30-35	30-35	1 hr. 5 min.
Week 4 *(easy)*	20-30	20-30	1 hr. 15 min.
Week 5	30-35	30-35	1 hr. 30 min.
Week 6	30-35	30-35	1 hr. 45 min.
Week 7	30-35	30-35	2 hours
Week 8 *(easy)*	20-30	20-30	60 *hills*
Week 9	30-35	30-35 *hills*	2 hrs. 30 min.
Week 10 *(easy)*	20-30	20-30	60 *hills*
Week 11	30-35	30-35 *hills*	60
Week 12	30-35	30-35	*HALF-MARATHON*

Training Notes:

_____

_____

_____

_____

_____

The Marathon Program

Mileage-Based Training

	Day One (run or cruise)		Day Two (run or cruise)		Weekend (cruise 10:2 or 20:3)	
	MILES	TIME	MILES	TIME	MILES	TIME
Week 1	3		3		4	
Week 2	3		3		5	
Week 3	3		3		6	
Week 4	3		3		7	
Week 5	3		3		8	
Week 6	3		3		9	
Week 7	3		3		10	
Week 8	3		3		6	
Week 9	3		3		12	
Week 10	3		3		6	
Week 11	3		3		6 hills	
Week 12	3 hills		3		14	
Week 13	2-3		2-3		6 hills	
Week 14	3		3		6 hills	
Week 15	3 hills		3		16-18	
Week 16	2-3		2-3		6 hills	
Week 17	3		3		6 hills	
Week 18	3 hills		3		18-20	
Week 19	2-3		2-3		6 hills	
Week 20	3		3		6 hills	
Week 21	3		3		20-22	
Week 22	2-3		2-3		6	
Week 23	3		3		6	
Week 24	3		3		26.2	

The Marathon Program

Time-Based Training

	Day One (run or cruise)	Day Two (run or cruise)	Weekend (cruise 10:2 or 20:3)
	TIME (minutes)	TIME (minutes)	TIME (hrs./min.)
Week 1	30-35	30-35	45
Week 2	30-35	30-35	55
Week 3	30-35	30-35	1 hr. 5 min.
Week 4	30-35	30-35	1 hr. 15 min.
Week 5	30-35	30-35	1 hr. 30 min.
Week 6	30-35	30-35	1 hr. 45 min.
Week 7	30-35	30-35	2 hours
Week 8	30-35	30-35	60 min.
Week 9	30-35	30-35	2 hrs. 30 min
Week 10	30-35	30-35	60 min.
Week 11	30-35	30-35	*60* min. (hills)
Week 12	30-35 *hills*	30-35	3 hours
Week 13	20-30	20-30	60 min (hills)
Week 14	30-35	30-35	60 min.
Week 15	30-35 *hills*	30-35	16-18
Week 16	20-30	20-30	60 min. (hills)
Week 17	30-35	30-35	60 min.
Week 18	30-35 *hills*	30-35	4 hours - then walk 30 minutes
Week 19	20-30	20-30	60 min. (hills)
Week 20	30-35	30-35	60 min.
Week 21	30-35	30-35	4 hrs. 30 min. then walk 30 minutes
Week 22	20-30	20-30	60 min.
Week 23	30-35	30-35	60 min.
Week 24	30-35	30-35	MARATHON

Index

Order Form

Corona House Publishing
P.O. Box 398
Manhattan Beach, CA 90267-0398, USA
Tel: (310) 546-6629 Fax: (310) 796-5774
E-mail: coronahouse@earthlink.net

Just Cruising: Simple Fitness for Busy People by Sue Ward, $12.95	$
California residents add 8.25% sales tax	$
Shipping (Standard Mail): $2.00 per book	$
Shipping (Priority Mail): $4.00 first two books, $2.00 each additional	$
TOTAL AMOUNT ENCLOSED (U.S. FUNDS)	$

Name:_____

Address:_____

_____

City, State:_____

Zip Code:_____

Phone:_____

E-mail:_____

Visit us at
www.coronahousepublishing.com

Order Form

Corona House Publishing
P.O. Box 398
Manhattan Beach, CA 90267-0398, USA
Tel: (310) 546-6629 Fax: (310) 796-5774
E-mail: coronahouse@earthlink.net

Just Cruising: Simple Fitness for Busy People by Sue Ward, $12.95 $

California residents add 8.25% sales tax $

Shipping (Standard Mail): $2.00 per book $

Shipping (Priority Mail): $4.00 first two books, $2.00 each additional $

TOTAL AMOUNT ENCLOSED (U.S. FUNDS) $

Name:_____

Address:_____

_____

City, State:_____

Zip Code:_____

Phone:_____

E-mail:_____

Visit us at
www.coronahousepublishing.com